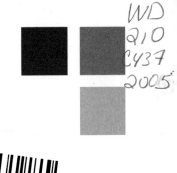

# The Challenges of Caring

# for the Obese Patient

Susan Gallagher, RN, MSN, MA, CWOCN, PhD

Matrix Medical Communications
*Edgemont, Pennsylvania*

*The Challenges of Caring for the Obese Patient*

Copyright © 2005 Matrix Medical Communications

*For information address:*

Matrix Medical Communications
4975 West Chester Pike
Suite 201
PO Box 445
Edgemont, PA 19028-0445

President/Group Publisher: Robert L. Dougherty
Partner: Patrick Scullin
Executive Editor: Elizabeth A. Klumpp
Associate Editor: Colleen M. Hutchinson
Sales Manager: J. Gregory Francis

Printed in the United States.

ISBN 0-9768526-0-8

This book contains photos and case report excerpts courtesy of SizeWise Rentals, Kansas City, Missouri.

Chapter 6 adapted with permission from Saxe Healthcare Communications. Gallagher SG. Obesity, the lungs, and airway management. *Perspectives* 2005;6(1):4–8.

**Note from the publisher:** *This book provides basic information about a broad range of medical conditions. It is not intended to serve as a tool for diagnosing illness, in prescribing treatments, or as a substitute for the physician/patient relationship. All persons concerned about medical symptoms or the possibility of disease are encouraged to seek professional care from an appropripate healthcare provider.*

# Dedication

To my father who taught me the meaning of perseverance, to Shannon who taught me the meaning of love, and to Doug who taught me the meaning of joy...*to each of you, thank you for enriching my world*

# Contents

# Overview

The word *obesity* originates from the Latin language and refers simply to the state of becoming "fattened by eating." *Bariatrics* is a term derived from the Greek word "baros," and is used today to refer to the practice of healthcare relating to the treatment of obesity and associated conditions. Issues related to weight hold public interest for several reasons. Certainly health and health-related concerns are important, as are demands for additional and specialized health services and overall increase in health costs.[1] The specialty of bariatrics is more and more important as the number of obese and overweight Americans is increasing. This is likely due to the dramatic physical, emotional, and economic costs of obesity.

The economic burden of obesity is significant with estimates of the total economic costs associated with the disease reaching 5.5 to 7.8 percent of all national healthcare expenditures.[2,3] Obesity is found to be associated with a 36-percent increase in inpatient and outpatient spending and a 28-percent increase in medications for obese smokers.[4] Obesity-related issues cost Americans nearly $150 billion annually; $117 billion is spent on health and health-related issues; another $33 billion is spent on the largely unsuccessful weight loss industry.

Overweight and obesity are common health conditions, and their prevalence is increasing nationally and globally. Recent estimates suggest that over 67 percent of adults in the US are overweight. Of all Americans between the ages of 26 and 75, 10 to 25 percent are obese, 130 million are overweight, and over nine million are morbidly obese. From 1976 to 2000, obesity increased from 14.4 percent to 30.9 percent. This increase has occurred regardless of age, gender, ethnicity, socioeconomic status, or race. To fully understand the meaning of these statistics, it is important to know how overweight and obesity are defined and measured.

Overweight refers to an excess of body weight compared to set standards. The excess weight may come from muscle, bone, fat, and/or water. Obesity refers specifically to the abnormal proportion of body fat. One can be overweight without being obese, as in the example of the body builder or other athlete who has greater than average muscle mass. However, many people who are overweight are

also obese. Both obese and overweight are quantitatively defined using body mass index (BMI).[5]

BMI is the most common and widely acceptable method of measuring overweight and obesity. BMI, which describes relative weight for height, is significantly correlated with total body fat content (Table 1). BMI is used to assess obesity; however, caution must be used when interpreting BMI in a child or a patient with edema, or ascites, in pregnant women, or in persons who are highly muscular, as an elevated BMI will not accurately reflect excess adiposity in these instances. Normal BMI falls in the range of 18.5 to 24.9. A patient with a BMI of >25 is considered overweight. Within the obese classification are grades I (BMI >30), II (BMI >35), and III (BMI >40).

Calculating BMI is relatively simple and inexpensive (See Table One: Calculating Body Mass Index). BMI is a mathematical formula based on height and weight, which assigns a certain number to an individual's relative risk for morbidity and mortality. This assessment tool is not gender specific. BMI is the measurement of choice for many obesity researchers, health professionals, and the popular press. Many health organizations, including policy makers, use BMI to measure and define

obesity and to establish criteria for certain procedures.[4] However, BMI as an assessment tool does carry certain limitations. One problem with using BMI as a measurement tool is that very muscular people may fall into the category of overweight when, in fact, they are very physically fit. Additionally, people who have lost large amounts of muscle mass may be in the healthy category when they actually have diminished nutritional reserves. Therefore, BMI has been most useful in tracking trends in the general population, and must be used with other assessment criteria when used to determine the health status of an individual patient.

In 1995, the World Health Organization (WHO) recommended using BMI to establish three grades or levels of overweight with the cutoff points of 25, 30, and 40. Two organizations within the National Institutes of Health (NIH)- the National Heart, Lung, and Blood Institute and the National Institutes of Diabetes, Digestive, and Kidney Diseases- concurred with this system, with the caveat that cutoff points are only a guide for definition and useful for comparative purposes across populations over time. For example, an overweight individual with a BMI of 29 does not instantly acquire all of the health consequences of obesity after crossing the threshold of BMI 30. However, researchers agree that health risks increase gradually as BMI increases.

The value of standardized measurement and definition is that all stakeholders are speaking the same language. Reimbursement guidelines and protocols may be defined by these standardized assessment tools. Like BMI, some tools are based on mathematical calculations of the relationship between height and weight, while others are based on measurements of body fat. Other assessment tools establish certain risk factors for comorbidities, such as the waist to hip ratio. For example, studies suggest that individuals with a high waist to hip ratio[6] are at risk for certain metabolic disorders, and the presence of obesity exacts greater tolls on this segment of the population.

Over a decade ago, the National Institutes of Health Consensus Development Conference on Gastrointestinal Surgery for Severe Obesity brought together surgeons, gastroenterologists, endocrinologists, psychiatrists, nutritionists, and other healthcare professionals, as well as the public, to address treatment options for severe obesity.[7] The NIH findings suggest that for morbidly obese people who have failed to lose weight using traditional methods and for whom obesity poses serious

---

**TABLE 1: CALCULATING BODY MASS INDEX**

**B**ody mass index (BMI) can be used to measure both overweight and obesity in adults. BMI does not directly measure percent of body fat, but it provides a more accurate measure of overweight and obesity than relying on weight alone. BMI is found by dividing a person's weight by height in meters squared. See www.nhlbisupport.com/bmi for a BMI calculator. The mathematical formula is: weight(kg)/height squared (m²)

**NIDDK. Statistics related to overweight and obesity. Accessed at: www.niddk.nih.gov**

---

medical and psychological risks, surgery is considered an effective treatment. For example, patients with a BMI of 40 or a BMI of 35, in the presence of comorbidities, are considered candidates who might benefit from bariatric weight loss surgery. The NIH guidelines continue to provide the standards and recommendations for bariatric weight loss surgery.

With the increasing numbers of adults and adolescents affected by obesity, it is likely that the number of patients having surgery will continue to increase, as current weight loss options seldom provide long-term weight loss.

From a historic perspective, bariatric weight loss surgery was first performed in the mid-twentieth century. This was largely due to the clinical observation that patients having the BillRoth II seemed to lose weight postoperatively. This sparked interest in a surgical approach to weight loss.

Two main categories of surgery are used to treat morbid obesity. These are gastric restrictive and combined gastric restriction and malabsorption. With gastric restriction, the size and capacity of the stomach are limited. The stomach pouch is often reduced to 15 to 30 milliliters. The Roux-en-Y gastric bypass (RYGB) is the most common procedure today, and combines gastric restriction and malabsorption by creating a small stomach pouch and bypassing 90 percent of the stomach, the duodenum, and a limb of jejunum of varying length. The RYGB reduces the capacity of the stomach so that the person eats less. It also reduces the absorption of calories contained in the food consumed.[7]

Excess body weight is a threat to health because it is associated with an increase of cardiovascular disease, type 2 diabetes, hypertension, infertility, stroke, hyperlipidemia, degenerative joint disease, gall stones, and some types of cancers.[8] When hospitalized, clinicians must recognize that most very overweight patients are at risk for certain hazards of immobility. Common immobility-related complications could include skin breakdown, cardiac deconditioning, deep vein thrombosis, muscle atrophy, urinary stasis, constipation, pain management challenges, and depression. Immobility also contributes to pulmonary complications such as atelectasis, pneumonia, delayed or traumatic intubation, and exacerbates pre-existing conditions such as overweight hypoventilation syndrome or sleep apnea. The obese patient is more inclined to develop complications resulting from a long hospitalization.

Several metabolic patterns of obesity exist. Android or abdominal obesity and excess visceral fat typically occur in men. Android obesity is associated with other metabolic conditions such as hypertension, insulin resistant type 2 diabetes mellitus, hyperuremia, and dyslipoprotemia, all of which comprise the condition known as Syndrome X. Therefore, the metabolic syndrome known as Syndrome X is not a disease; rather it is a group of conditions that are important warning signs that serve as predictors of heart disease and diabetes.[8]

Visceral fat obesity results in increased waist to hip ratio of fat distribution, expressing a mutation of the beta three-adrenoreceptor gene. The mechanism may be enhanced sensitivity to catecholamine-mediated lipolysis, and is associated with glucose intolerance (type 2 diabetes mellitus) and hypertension. Gynecoid obesity typically occurs among females and is manifested with fat deposits in the hips, buttocks, and upper legs. There is less metabolic significance in gynecoid obesity.

The National Institutes of Health describes obesity as a complex and multifactorial condition. However, regardless of the etiology, it is often considered simply a condition of excess energy stores in the form of fat.[9] Some of the common etiologies that influence this balance are thought to be related to emotional and environment issues, genetics, medication and others. Some contend that prejudice and discrimination aimed at larger people fuels emotional issues that lead to further threat of weight and weight concerns. Prejudice and discrimination exist in employment, health care, education, public places, and housing, to name a few.[10]

Environmental etiologies are closely related to nutrition, activity, and physical trauma.[11] From a nutritional perspective, even before the child is born,

## THE GASTRIC PACEMAKER

People wanting to lose weight may soon be in for a shock! Researchers at the University of Pennsylvania and eight other medical centers are conducting a two-year trial with over 200 patients. The study is expected to conclude in mid-2006. Transneuronix Inc. of Mount Arlington, New Jersey, which has developed the gastric pacemaker, hopes results from the trial will lead to FDA approval. The experimental device is a battery-operated electrical generator about the size of a pocket watch and is surgically implanted in the abdomen, with two wires connecting to the stomach wall. In a similar way that a pacemaker sends electrical impulses to the heart, the experimental gastric pacemaker sends a small current to the stomach through four electrodes on the wires. The electrical current is activated, adjusted, or monitored by a handheld computer in the doctor's office that communicates to the pacemaker through a radio signal. Interestingly, patients report they cannot feel the impulse. To date, it is unclear how the device really works. Some speculate that it causes the stomach to relax and signal a feeling of fullness. Others contend it may simply send a message of satiety to the brain. Regardless, this may be an option for the future.

the mother's nutrition plays a part in the child's predisposition toward obesity, as intrauterine over or under nutrition can lead to weight issues. Infant feeding further creates this predisposition. The commonly consumed American diet is largely high-fat, low-protein, highly processed, comprised of frequent large meals/snacks and highly sugared drinks, often supersized. As of 1997, 46 percent of family food expenditures were spent on meals outside the home, with 34 percent of the total food dollars spent on fast foods. Inactivity is largely due to dramatic lifestyle changes, which are likely a result of television and Internet, urban lifestyles, and labor saving devices.

Some ethnic groups are predisposed to obesity by what has been described as the "thrifty gene." This theory proposed in 1962 by James Neel helps explain why many Pima Indians are overweight. Neel's theory is based on the fact that for thousands of years groups that relied on farming, hunting, and fishing endured prolonged periods of feast and alternatively famine. These groups were thought to adapt to these changes by developing a thrifty gene that allowed for fat storage in times of feast, and protected them in times of famine. This adaptation was useful as long as famine existed, but

adjusting to the typical Western lifestyle has been problematic for the Pima Indians, contributing to high levels of body fat.[12]

A genetic predisposition accounts for 80 percent of the risk for obesity. Obese children with obese parents are more likely to have genetic-related disorders linked to obesity than are obese children of thin parents. A child of two obese parents has an 80 percent chance of becoming an obese adult, and a child of two normal weighted parents has a 15 percent chance of becoming obese.

Several rare genetic conditions can lead to obesity, including: Prader-Willi, Lawrence-Moon, and Bardet-Biedl Syndrome(s). Additionally, other chromosomal defects lead to leptin deficiencies, adipocyte complement-related protein (Acrp30) deficiencies, and appetite hormone abnormalities. Genetic problems can lead to a susceptibility to environmental factors, which can include: density of taste receptors on the tongue, serotonin transporter gene polymorphism, and dopamine-receptor gene abnormalities.

Sixty-six percent of obese people suffer from osteoarthritis. Osteoarthritis is a degenerative skeletal condition that worsens with weight gain. Those individuals with a BMI

greater than 40 are significantly at risk for disability associated with arthritis.[13] Functional impairment and musculoskeletal pain interfere with activities of daily living and therefore limited activity leads to an increase in weight gain. However, a healthy weight is essential to treatment and prevention because it helps reduce stress on joints.[14]

Hyperkinetic circulation, with increased blood flow, occurs more frequently among patients with a greater body mass. Hyperkinetic circulation may cause overperfusion of tissues, which the body responds to with vasoconstriction. Consequently, this increase in total peripheral resistance leads to arterial hypertension.

Congestive heart failure occurs from increased systemic arterial pressure—high blood pressure. Fluid overload is due to edema from right sided failure, which is the result of increased pulmonary artery pressures, prolonged QT intervals, and sudden death from tachydysrhythmias.

Respiratory compromise is manifested by elevated intra-abdominal pressure, reductions in lung volumes, and decreased muscle endurance. An increased oxygen demand, hypoventilation, and hypercapnia, sleep apnea, and sudden death are not uncommon. Obstructive sleep apnea

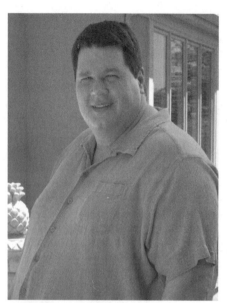

**Regardless of the etiologies of the patient's obesity, health care providers best serve the larger, heavier person when there is an understanding of the complex clinical needs of the patient.**

affects 10 to 20 percent of obese individuals.

Endocrine changes typically include: elevated plasma rennin and the aldosterone levels in the presence or absence of hypertension, elevated levels of atrial natriuretic factor, which causes elevated volume and high blood pressure, and Syndrome X. Syndrome X is a phenomenon which is initially characterized by hyperinsulinemia, and later insulin resistance. Syndrome X is associated with central or visceral obesity, an android or male fat distribution, and has more serious metabolic consequences.

Intra-abdominal pressure is a widespread condition among morbidly obese people. It is best described as an increased pressure related to creating intra-abdominal compartment syndrome. This condition can lead to Bartlett's esophagitis, which is a risk factor for esophageal cancer. Stress urinary incontinence, varicose veins, hemorrhoids, and abdominal hernias can occur. Fatty liver leading to liver fibrosis, nephrosis from low renal flow rates, and pseudotumor cerebri can develop. Some contend that elevated intra-abdominal pressure can lead to wound separation.

The skin is affected in many ways. Pressure ulcers, candidiasis, delayed wound healing, incontinence dermatitis, and irritation in the intertriginous areas are common, especially in the presence of comorbidities and immobility.

Psychological consequences of obesity can develop; however, it is important to recognize that when comparing obese and non-obese people for mental health conditions, the only condition seen consistently more frequently among obese people is situational depres-

sion. Prejudice and discrimination are thought to contribute to this situational depression. Children as young as six years old have been found to label silhouettes designed to look like obese people as "lazy, dirty, stupid, ugly, and cheats." College acceptance, employment, advances, and other opportunities have been lost as a result of the applicant's size or weight.

Up to 30 percent of obese people experience one or more types of depression. Being female and having an eating disorder places a person at greater risk for depression. The greater the person's BMI, the more likely situational depression will occur, and once weight occurs, the incidence of depression decreases. For example, 40 to 90 percent of severely obese people are thought to be depressed.[15] Many overweight and obese people express body image dissatisfaction, viewing their bodies with hostility and discontent, describing themselves as ugly and despicable. Size acceptance groups work diligently with larger people to help them understand their unique body and come to terms with the value and contribution each person makes as a holistic person, irrespective of body size or weight. Although controversial, some research supports the theory that obese people have experienced a higher degree of psychological trauma; some studies suggest that 25 percent of obese people have experienced sexual, physical, or verbal abuse as compared to 6 percent in nonobese people.

## SUMMARY

Regardless of the etiologies of the patient's obesity, health care providers best serve the larger, heavier person when there is an understanding of the complex clinical needs of the patient. At every level, discipline, and service provided, considerations need to be made for size and weight. Measures need to be taken to provide safe care, which protects both the patient and caregiver.

## REFERENCES

1.  Weighing in on obesity. Grantmakers in health, Brief 11. Washington DC.
2.  Kort MA, Langley PC, Cox ER. A review of cost-of-illness studies on obesity. *Clinical Therapy* 1998;20:772–9.
3.  Thompson D, Wolf AM. The medical cost burden of obesity. *Obesity Review* 2001;2:189–97.
4.  Strum R. The effects of obesity, smoking, and drinking on medical problems and costs. *Health Affairs* 220;21:245–53.
5.  NIDDK. Statistics related to overweight and obesity. Accessed at: http://www.niddk.nih.gov.
6.  Gallagher S, Langlois C, Spacht D, Blackett A, Henns T. Preplanning with protocols for skin and wound care in obese patients. *Advances in Skin and Wound Care* 2004;17:436–41.
7.  Gallagher S. Taking the weight off with bariatric surgery. *Nursing* 2005;34:58–64.
8.  What is Syndrome X? Accessed at: http://pritikin.com/eperspective/jan-feb05/0501_02.htm.
9.  National Institutes of Health. Clinical guidelines on the identification, evaluation, and treatment of overweight and obesity in adults. *Obesity Research* 1998;6:51s–209s.
10. Puhl R & Brownell K. Bias, discrimination and obesity. *Obesity Research* 2001;9:788–803.
11. Falkner NH, Neumarksztainer D, Story M, et al. Social, educational, psychological correlates of weight status in adolescents. *Obesity Research* 2001;9:32–42.
12. Obesity and diabetes. Accessed at: http://diabetes.niddk.nih.gov/dm/pubs/pima/obesity/obesity.htm.
13. Okoro CA, Hootman JM, Strine TW, et al. Disability, arthritis, and body weight among adults 45 years and older. *Obesity Research* 2004;12:854–861.
14. Obesity Today and Tomorrow. Accessed at: http://www.arthritis.org/communities/nychapter/advocacynews/advocacy_summer2004.asp.
15. Pine D, Rise B, Goldstein SW, et al. The association between childhood depression and adult body mass index. *Pediatrics* 2001;107:1049–56.

# Childhood Obesity

**2**

**M**ore than 60 percent of eight-year-old girls are dieting. Many think they are overweight; 90 percent are not. Affluent toddlers have shown failure to thrive because their parents, fearing fat offspring, underfed them. Unfortunately, parents' concerns may be very real. For example, in studies of first graders, overweight children were selected less often as friends and teammates.[1] Last year a young boy shot and killed a fellow student who constantly harassed him because of his weight. And in the past two years, two young boys shot and killed themselves because of their weight.[2]

Obesity and overweight are the most common health problems facing US children today.[3] Twenty-five percent of adolescents are thought to be overweight. Since 1971, the number of overweight children has more than doubled for children ages 6 to 11 and more than tripled for children ages 12 to 19.[4] The health burden placed on children who are overweight is considerable. Common medical complications include hypertension, type II diabetes

**CRITERIA FOR ADOLESCENT BARIATRIC WEIGHT LOSS SURGERY**

- **Attained physical maturity**
- **Failed medically supervised weight loss efforts**
- **BMI >40 with serious comorbidities or >50 with comorbidities**
- **Emotional maturity to commit to lifelong lifestyle changes**
- **Agree to avoid pregnancy for one year postoperatively**
- **Demonstrate capacity to provide informed consent**
- **Supportive family environment**

**For more detailed description and discussion see: Inge T, Krebs NF, Garcia VF, et al. Surgery for severely overweight adolescents: Concerns and recommendations, *Pediatrics* 2004:114(7):217–23.**

mellitus, respiratory concerns, and depression. In addition, an overweight adolescent tends to become an overweight adult.[5] Living with obesity is extremely difficult for anyone, especially an adolescent. Etiologies, trends to address the issues, the cultural meaning of obesity, and challenges in caring for a very large child are presented. This emerging public health crisis is described with examples of hospital and community-based intervention.

## ADDRESSING THE ISSUES

In response to this alarming data, the media is spending more time than ever trying to define the problem and explore areas of interest to consumers. Parents, communities, and policymakers are actively seeking strategies to make changes. From a legislative perspective, two bills specifically addressing childhood obesity are before

Congress. Senate Bill 2551 "Childhood Obesity Reduction Act" was introduced June 21, 2004, by Senators Bill Frist R-TN and Ron Wyden D-OR. A similar bill with the same title was introduced into the House of Representatives HR 4941 on July 22, 2004, by Congresswoman Kay Granger R-TX and Congressman Steny Hoyer D-MD. Both bills are directed toward schools and school districts. Still other bills are seeking to form a Congressional Council on Childhood Obesity. The goal of the Council is to encourage early elementary school and middle schools to develop and implement plans to reduce or prevent obesity, promote healthy nutritional choices, increase physical activity, and provide information to secondary schools. Other notable bills before Congress include S1428 Commonsense Consumption Act HR2227 Obesity

Prevention Act, S1172 IMPACT, S1201 YMCA Healthy Teen Act, and HR 2024 Medicaid Obesity Treatment Act (See Access Legislative Efforts). Each effort for change best serves children when created to promote physical and emotional health and well being. This is hard to do without an understanding of the cultural meaning of obesity and the barriers it creates.

## THE CULTURAL MEANING OF WEIGHT

The cultural significance of weight and weight-related issues affects everyone, but perhaps children most of all. Conversation surrounding issues of weight prevail in lunchrooms, buses, social events, and schools. This comes at a time when women are heavier than ever. For example, in 1991, an average woman in her twenties weighed 142 pounds, compared to 155 pounds today. And a woman in her thirties weighed 154 pounds in 1991 as compared to 167 now.

Consider an ongoing survey conducted by *Glamour* magazine. In 1984, the magazine conducted its first survey pertaining to women and their bodies. At that time, 41 percent of women were reportedly unhappy with their bodies primarily because of weight issues. In 1998, body confidence level dipped as 53 percent of women said they were unhappy with their appearance; 44 percent admitted to starving to lose weight; 17 percent had tried vomiting, and 35 percent used liquid diets. Today, the statistics closely reflect the 1998 findings with just a few positive changes: only 10 percent of women have resorted to vomiting, and 83 percent say they'd rather be slightly heavy and healthy than thin and unhealthy. However, Kelly Brownell, Director of the Center for Eating and Weight Disorders at Yale University, explains that even thin isn't enough anymore. "In the 60s and 70s, the pressure was just to be very thin, but today superimposed on that is the need to be contoured and sculpted." Despite the imperative to thin and contoured bodies, Americans are heavier than ever. This preoccupation with body appearance is continuing to increase. It makes sense that this preoccupation affects our children and adolescents in their attitudes and the attitudes of their parents and other influential adults.

## ETIOLOGIES AND THE FAMILY

Overweight and obesity among children and adolescents is generally thought to be caused by a genetic predisposition, lack of physical activity, unhealthy eating patterns,

or a combination of these factors. More specifically, overweight and obesity are closely related to technological, social, economic, and environmental changes that have reduced physical activity and increased food access and passive energy consumption. Increases in sedentary activities, such as video games and television, decrease in physical activity because of safety or time constraints, and an increase of high fat and high energy foods are likely to play a critical factor in the current trend.[6]

Regardless of the etiologies of obesity in childhood and adolescence, childhood obesity leads to approximately 30 percent of adult obesity. Adults who are obese as children have more severe obesity. In addressing causality, various theories and studies targeting prenatal, genetic, familial, or environmental factors are important. For example, family factors clearly influence the prevalence of obesity in children. A major risk factor for obesity in children is parental obesity. A child has an 80-per-

cent chance of being obese when both parents are obese, and a 40-percent chance when only one parent is obese. When neither parent is obese, chances of childhood obesity are reduced to seven percent. This may not only be genetic, but may also be due to family influences on the health of its members.

The family shapes the child's early lifestyle and habits, and many experts place blame on television viewing and other sedentary activities. For example, the average US high school graduate will have spent 18,000 hours in front of a television set and 12,000 hours in school. This doesn't even account for time spent watching videotapes, playing video or computer games, or surfing the Internet, which when added to TV viewing averages six and a half hours daily. Notably, the average American lives within one and one-half miles from a public park. Regardless, a growing body of research suggests that the more television kids watch, the more likely they are to be

**WEBSOURCES**

- **Johnson C. Raising Largely Positive Kids. Available at: www.radiancemagazine.com/issues/1999/fall99_kids.htm.**

- **Summer N & Rodgveller C. Interpreting size bias: A summary of the Kids Come in All Sizes workshop, Available at: www.cswd.org/kidsandcrart.html.**

overweight. In fact, the average child views television 4 to 5 hours daily, and over one-third view over five hours daily. Researchers at Harvard University found that children who view more than five hours of television a day are nearly five times more likely to be overweight than their peers who view two hours a day or less.[7] To compound this dilemma, 25 percent of a child's food intake occurs in front of a television.[8]

The family establishes norms that guide decision making not only in relation to activity, but other areas as well. For example, problem solving skills are learned behaviors, and the family serves as the mentor for acquiring these skills. Other family influences include body weight and adiposity of family members, as well as eating and activity habits. Additionally, parenting influences the child's long-term health habits. Parents serve as role models for appropriate behaviors pertaining to care and respect for the body. But more importantly, the family influences a social learning environment. Lessons learned can lead to a healthy or unhealthy understanding of weight and health, depending on understandings held by family members. During childhood, young people are socialized to the importance of physical appearance.

**SHAPEDOWN PEDIATRIC OBESITY PROGRAM**

**The program was developed by a dietitian with interdisciplinary input. This family-centered approach recognizes skills of body and spirit including nurturing, limit setting, nutrition, activity, and good health. By the tenth week, the children are having activity five times a week, and a minimum of 1,200 calories per day is required. Maintenance is a 20-week program with a minimum of a one-year tune-up session. Staff members complete a 46-hour training period. For more information please contact: shapedown@aol.com.**

There is a critical relationship between body image and self-concept. Dissatisfaction has been evident in both girls and boys who perceive themselves different from the norm. The normal developmental patterns intended for children, which are establishing relationships and becoming comfortable with one's body and independence, coupled with the stigma of overweight and obesity, can lead to eating disorders and subsequent nutritional and developmental deficiencies.

## UNDERSTANDING CHANGE

Heavier children continue to struggle with issues of self-worth, body image, and self-esteem. They continue to suffer from peer rejection because of their body size and shape. Most teachers don't know what to do, and neither do parents and other stakeholders. The challenge is to promote a healthy lifestyle while preventing an abnormal preoccupation with physical appearance, the body, and food. Supportive information on how to help

children lead happy, healthy lives at whatever size they are meant to be must be communicated to parents, caregivers, teachers, health professionals, and policymakers.[9] A key clinical role is to explain the concept of making changes within the family. Parents, other key adults. and older children best serve the needs of an obese child by being supportive and should never make fun of or allow others to make fun of the child. In cases where the child must lose weight for health reasons, clinicians should provide parents with the tools to explain the need for weight loss to the child. Clinicians should encourage parents to serve as role models for a healthier lifestyle.

Remind parents to implement the same healthy diet for the entire family, not just select individuals. Review with parents the concept of the food pyramid, consisting of carbohydrates, proteins, fats, vitamins, and minerals because they often do not fully understand the meaning of a balanced nutritional diet. Encourage parents to reduce fatty food and empty calories, such as sweets and processed snacks, leaving healthy snacks in an area easily accessible to the child. Healthy snacks might include fruits, vegetables, yogurt, and unsweetened cereals. Remind parents to avoid using food as a reward or the lack of food as a punishment. Teach the child to appreciate healthy meals by involvement in meal preparation. Don't allow kids to eat in front of the TV; this makes a bad habit of associating eating with TV. Eat in an unrushed setting as a family. Teach the child what foods to buy when eating away from home. Kids love fast food but they also like variety in their menu. Parents can improve and invent healthy meals. Emphasize the value of vegetables.

Encourage parents to get exercise as a family because it promotes physical and social development. Plan special active family outings, such as hiking or playing at the park. Assign household tasks to every family member and routinely vary responsibility to prevent boredom with certain activities. Parents should consider enrolling their children in structured community or school activities.

Understanding childhood obesity and the methods available for managing this condition become increasingly more important. Some children will fail at weight loss regardless of efforts. Stakeholders have begun to examine bariatric weight loss surgery as one tool in helping children, primarily adolescents, address issues of weight. One hundred forty-four thousand adults had bariatric weight loss surgery in 2004. Across the country, centers are offering bariatric weight loss surgery to those under 18 years of age. This poses a number of moral questions.

## THE UNSETTLING QUESTIONS: AN ETHICAL DISCUSSION

With more bariatric weight loss centers offering surgery as a treatment option to younger patients, it is time to consider the way we address the hard choices in caring for complex, vulnerable populations. Childhood obesity is painful emotionally, carrying serious physical consequences. The recent introduction of surgery to the "tool box" of treatment options poses numerous ethical questions. How do we decide? This controversy raises more questions than answers.

Ethics is defined as the philosophic study of right and wrong action of a moral nature. An ethical dilemma occurs when two or more unacceptable choices exist concerning a problem of a moral nature, and a decision must be made between these choices. In healthcare settings, this is especially tragic in that the "right" choice may still hold significant pain and suffering. Using an ethical framework to determine the best choice is thought to reduce the amount of pain and suffering that can occur but still is not a guarantee. This is why ethical debate is so disturbing. By nature, healthcare clinicians want what is best for their patients, and even though models are available to frame ethical questions, there is no science to ensure protection of our vulnerable patients. Childhood obesity is one of those areas that pose numerous ethical challenges, and the debate pertaining to bariatric weight loss surgery is intense and heated in many cases, posing a significant ethical dilemma.

Consider the Corrigan case. When 13-year-old Christina Corrigan died of congestive heart failure in her home, she weighed 680 pounds. Her thighs were 54 inches in circumference, and her calves were 47 inches around. It was reported she was covered with bedsores. She had been to the physician 99 times. What happened in this situation? In retrospect, judgments can be made as to the options for managing this type of heartbreaking situation. But the reality in these complex circumstances is that numerous unacceptable choices existed, and the challenge to all stakeholders involved was to choose the least unacceptable choice. The questions pertaining to this case revolve around responsibility/culpability. And when we consider childhood obesity, the entire community becomes involved in the debate.

Some of the ethical questions posed by this situation are as follows:

1. To what extent is Child Protective Services responsible to intervene on the part of children who are seriously at risk for health consequences related to excessive body weight?
2. What is the responsibility of healthcare providers when faced with a child whose health and life are seriously at risk because of excess body weight?
3. What is the responsibility of a parent(s) when their child's weight poses serious health and social consequences?
4. To what extent is a parent(s) culpable for the death of a child when/if social institutes fail?

Although each of these questions is important, for purposes of this discussion, number 2 poses the most profound frame for debate among healthcare professionals. Christina's body mass index (BMI) was 139, with healthy defined as 21 to 25. The first step in an ethical analysis is collecting the data that is available. In Christina's case, most clinicians want to know what medical exams and lab tests had been done. What occurred in those 99 physician visits? How did this child come to weigh 680 pounds? What was her diet? What activities did she engage in? When did she stop exercising? Did she go to school? Could she ride in a car? What kind of clothing could she wear? Was she able to shower in a standard shower stall? What treatment options were available or offered to her? Would bariatric weight loss surgery have been an option for this child? Is 680 pounds too heavy to safely perform the surgery? Is 13 years old too young?

The purpose of this case analysis is to begin a painful but essential dialogue concerning options available to our obese children, their parents, and the community. Remember, in ethical debate, there is no right choice. We, as healthcare professionals, work with patients and their families in making every effort to ensure the best choice based on the information provided to us at the time. With the recent introduction of pediatric bariatric weight loss surgery, we need to participate in lively debate pertaining to options in managing the complexities of this emotionally and physically vulnerable group. However, the reality is that ethics and ethical debate are often troubling because there is no right choice.[10]

## BARIATRIC WEIGHT LOSS SURGERY (BWLS)

Korsica Merrill is a 265-pound 14-year-old girl who decided the only way she could trim down was through bariatric weight loss surgery. The question raised was "Is a 14-year-old too young for a surgical procedure that would rearrange her digestive tract and reduce her stomach to the size of a golf ball?"

Fifteen-year-old Charles Fabrikant stopped going to sporting events because he couldn't fit into stadium seats. It was reported that although he loved playing baseball and basketball, he simply no longer was able to run and consequently stopped participating. Korsica and Charles both resorted to weight loss surgery after numerous unsuccessful attempts at weight control. Additionally, Korsica and

Charles each have a parent who had successfully lost weight and improved their quality of life after surgery. Three centers in the Chicago area perform weight loss surgery in the under-18 population. Dr. Jeffrey Rosen of the WISH Center was quoted saying, "Severely obese adolescents may be better off having the surgery now, while they are still healthy, instead of trying 20 years of diet and exercise." Dr. Frantzides, Korsica's surgeon, explains, "Obese adolescents often suffer from depression and low self esteem and are more likely to be ridiculed. They are scarred by psychological and mental abuse."[11]

Childhood obesity to date has not been designated as an illness, and therefore treatment options are limited in a reimbursement sense. Recent research suggests, however, that BWLS for the obese adolescent who suffers from functional impairment related to weight is a successful treatment option. Dr. Harvey Sugerman concurs, explaining that BWLS is a safe form of treatment with subsequent weight loss, with significant resolution of weight-related comorbidities, and improved self esteem and socialization.[12] Some experts contend that laparoscopic BWLS may serve as a safe alternative for the adolescent population who has

not responded to conventional weight loss efforts.[13] Perhaps most important to date is another study that examined the value of an interdisciplinary comprehensive weight management center within a children's hospital. The center involved in the study offered Roux-en-Y gastric bypass both laparoscopically and open. The study suggested that with the use of pediatric specialists, BWLS can be considered a safe alternative.[14] However, the key to this approach seems to indicate a need for proper preoperative preparation and postoperative followup.[15]

Not everyone so readily embraces this option. The National Association to Advance Fat Acceptance (NAAFA), founded in 1969, is a nonprofit human rights organization dedicated to ending discrimination based on body size. A press release was distributed by NAAFA wherein it was reported, "From Carnie Wilson's highly publicized Internet broadcast surgery to a recent CNN story, which documents the emergence of weight loss surgery for children, weight loss certainly garnered its share of media attention with a focus on the success stories." Representatives from NAAFA contend there are alternative treatments for obesity-related conditions. And one expert further expresses, "If you talk to people considering weight loss surgery, they often speak of being desperate to lose weight, but I often wonder if this desperation is caused by health considerations or by societal bias against fat people." NAAFA's official position is, "The psychosocial suffering that fat people face is more appropriately relieved by social and political reform than by surgery."[16]

Like NAAFA, the American Academy of Pediatrics (AAP) takes a conservative approach. However, instead of opposing the surgery entirely, AAP has established criteria to determine which adolescents might be considered for BWLS. Like other groups, both NAAFA and AAP strive to ensure safety emotionally and physically as it pertains to caring for children, a vulnerable, protected population. This should be the goal of individuals, institutions, communities, and public policymakers who hold an obligation to protect the interests of children.[17]

## SUMMARY

The challenge of loving, caring for, or teaching an overweight child can be emotionally overwhelming. To date, a number of common sense strategies have been helpful for some but not for all. Parents, communities, and policy makers are striving to develop methods to control obesity among the younger population.

## REFERENCES

1.  Frontline Fat 1998. PBS Publication 1998. Available at www.pbs.org.
2.  Kids Project. Available at: www.radiancemagazine.com/kids project/kids.html.
3.  Stauss RS, Pollack HA. Epidemic increase in childhood overweight, 1986–1998. *J Am Med Assoc* 2001:286:2845–8.
4.  *The role of media in childhood obesity.* Kaiser Family Foundation. Available at: www.kff.org.
5.  US Department of Health and Human Services. *The Surgeon General's Call to Action to prevent and decrease overweight and obesity.* Rockville, MD: US Department of Health and Human Services, Office of the Surgeon General. 2001.
6.  About childhood obesity. Available at: www.health.nsw.gov.au/obesity-summit/asult/about.html. Access date: January 2005.
7.  McAllister R. Tube time promotes childhood obesity. Available at: www.rallieon health.com.
8.  HealthTech. Obesity Management-Clinical Focus. December 2004. Available at: www.healthtech.org.
9.  Henry L. Childhood obesity: What can be done to help today's youth. *Pediatric Nursing* 2005;31:13–16.
10. Gallagher S. *A Tragic Case of Childhood Obesity.* Ann Arbor, MI: UMI Press, 2000.
11. Obese teens turn to surgery as a last resort. Available at: www.sun-times.com;. Access date: March, 2004
12. Sugerman HJ, Sugerman EL, DeMaria EJ, et al. Bariatric surgery for severely obese adolescents. *J Gastro Surg* 2003;7:102–7.
13. Stanford A, Glascock JM, Eid GM, et al. Laparoscopic Roux-en-Y gastric bypass in morbidly obese adolescents. *J Pediatric Surg* 2003;38:430–3.
14. Inge TH, Garcia V, Daniels S, et al. A multidisciplinary approach to adolescent bariatric surgery patient. *J Pediatric Surg* 2004;39:442–7.
15. Abu-Abeid S, Gavert N, Klausner JM, et al. Bariatric surgery in adolescence. *J Pediatric Surg* 2004;38:1379–82.
16. Kids and weight loss surgery. Available at: naafa.org/news/kid-sandwls. Access date: January 2005.
17. Gallagher S. Caring for the child who is obese: Mobility, caregiver safety, environmental accommodation, and legal concerns. *Pediatr Nurs* 2005;31:17–20.

**3**

# Bariatric Weight Loss Surgery

In the past decade, bariatric weight loss surgery (BWLS) has increased 644 percent. Despite questions pertaining to reimbursement, 160,000 to 180,000 people will have BWLS in the US in 2005, according to the American Society for Bariatric Surgery. Some experts feel these numbers are modest and that over 200,000 people will have BWLS in 2005. The reason may be because of the increasing awareness of mortality and morbidity related to obesity. For example, 400,000 Americans die prematurely from obesity-related complica-

tions. Obesity affects every organ of the body.[1] Many people having BWLS report trying hundreds of diet and exercise programs. Surgical management of obesity may be appropriate for as many as 10 million Americans who are considered morbidly obese. BWLS is aimed at controlling obesity, and its corresponding medical, physical, social, and psychological consequences.[2]

## CRITERIA FOR BWLS

Candidates for surgery must meet certain criteria. For example, the patient must have a

**THE VOICE OF THE PATIENT—THE POWER OF CHANGE**

My oldest sister was obese, with a BMI of 56. Ten years ago she was admitted to the hospital for fatigue and generalized pain. She delayed admission as long as she could. Therefore, she was very ill when she finally arrived at the hospital. There was difficulty making any type of diagnosis because she was too large for much of the diagnostic equipment. Throughout the hospitalization she had horrible pain. She died within 10 weeks, and to this day we don't know why. We believe the problem was two-fold. Certainly my sister's weight was at the heart of the problem, but secondly, we wanted to know why she could not be accommodated. Last week, my aunt had BWLS. What a difference. Clinical experts were everywhere asking, "How is your pain? Can we help you turn? Have you been out of bed?" And on and on. The staff was so proficient and confident in caring for her. I appreciate all of the changes. Our only regret is that if the interest in caring for larger people had started earlier, it might have saved my sister's life.

body mass index (BMI) of greater than 40kg/m$^2$, or greater than 35kg/m$^2$ with co-morbidities, such as sleep apnea, type 2 diabetes mellitus, hyperlipidemia, hypertension, or other significant weight-related comorbidity[3]. Before BWLS is considered for reimbursement, most insurance carriers require documentation of three unsuccessful attempts on medically-supervised weight loss programs. The patient will need a thorough physical exam, including health history and weight history. Screening must determine absence of physical or emotional disorders that might be at the heart of weight gain. The screening process also includes multiple evaluations to assess whether a patient will be able to comply

with the many lifelong changes that will be required postoperatively. Sometimes family members will be involved with this evaluation, as families can be a very important part of postoperative adaptation to change.

## COSTS OF OBESITY

Obesity is costly emotionally and economically, and the economic costs of obesity continue to climb.[4] In 2003, a report found that medical expenditures due to obesity averaged 5.3 percent, totally nearly $133 billion[5]. And the obese American aged 18 to 36 generates 36 percent more medical expenses than the nonobese.[6] Nearly half of the costs of obesity are paid out of tax supported health insurance. Twenty-one percent of elderly

Medicare patients were obese. Among the poor disabled Medicare recipients, 30 percent were obese.[7]

## THE GOAL OF BWLS

Patients' quality of life and health improve both short- and long-term following surgery.[8] Seventy-five percent of patients are expected to lose 75 to 80 percent of their excess body weight. Well over 70 to 80 percent of patients with hypertension will no longer require medications, and well over 90 percent of patients with type 2 diabetes are expected to be free of their medications. Sleep apnea, asthma, reflux, fatigue, and shortness of breath are drastically improved if not completely resolved. Bilevel positive airway pressure (BiPAP) for sleep apnea and other supportive devices may no longer be required within just months of surgery. Patients report an overall sense of well being. There is an expected reduction in the risks of heart disease, pulmonary disorders, and cancer. Patients can expect a significant improvement in quality of life and self esteem.[9]

## PATIENT TEACHING

Patient teaching is a collaborative effort between the patient, family, and the health care team, and should begin on first contact. Patients must understand that the surgery itself does not guarantee long-term weight management. Commitment to lifelong behavioral changes is essential to the success of this strategy. Patients will need instruction preoperatively and reinforcement of that instruction postoperatively. Patients will need to understand the importance of early ambulation to decrease the likelihood of developing deep venous thrombosis (DVT), pneumonia, or ileus. The patient needs to be instructed on the use and purpose of the incentive spirometer to prevent atelectasis/pneumonia, and to understand the rationale for oxygen and respiratory treatments, which promotes healing and prevent the risk of respiratory compromise. Pain management and medication administration should also be a focus of patient teaching. Various medications, dosages, and routes can be used and patient instructions should be tailored to fit their situation.[10]

Dietary teaching will vary according to facility and surgeon preference. A dietitian should be involved in the multidisciplinary approach to patient teaching. Each patient will need his or her own individualized dietary plan.

Wound care will vary based on type of surgery performed. A small adhesive bandage may be all that is necessary for a laparoscopic procedure. The left trochanteric site is at risk

for infection because it is most likely to have contamination from the internal organs to the skin surface. The patient should be reminded to report any unusual tenderness at the site. A dry dressing over the surgical site and drain sites will be used after an open procedure and will need to be changed daily and as needed.

Home health assistance may be necessary for patients if there is complicated wound care required. The patient needs to understand that discharge instructions will be provided and should include information about follow-up appointments, wound/dressing care, drain tube care, activity, diet, medications, and support groups. It is imperative that patients follow up with their primary care provider soon after discharge to ensure adjustments to medications

and procedures due to control of comorbidities.

The patient must understand the need to consume at least three meals daily, chewing food completely before swallowing. Liquids cannot be taken at meal times, and at the first indication of fullness the patient needs to stop eating. High calorie, sugar- and fat-dense foods and beverages need to be avoided. A daily chewable or liquid multivitamin with iron is important to supplement dietary intake. The patient must commit to daily activity of at least 30 minutes.

## PSYCHOLOGICAL EVALUATION

Despite meeting the weight criteria for BWLS, some patients will still not be candidates until underlying psychological issues are resolved. Preoperative psychological

---

**RESPIRATORY IDEAS**

Ten to twenty percent of obese patients have some level of respiratory dysfunction. Patients seem to breathe more easily when the bed is at 30 degrees as this reduces the weight of the abdominal adipose tissue and edema, which reportedly presses against the diaphragm. The patient may need encouragement to perform leg exercises and breathing and coughing exercises. Early activity is encouraged in that this decreases the chances of immobility-related complications. In addition, in the early postoperative period, patients may have an increased morbidity from surgery and anesthesia in the form of atelectasis, deep vein thrombosis and pulmonary embolus.[15] Sequential compression devices to accommodate the larger leg are available, to that extent foot "squeezers" are useful in that they usually better accommodate the larger patient. Full body rotation therapy is also a strategy in controlling for atelectasis in the postoperative patient who is limited in mobility.

evaluations are required by many insurance carriers, and are thought to serve as a predictor of the candidates' postoperative success in the face of long-term lifelong changes. Some BWLS programs and surgeons require a preoperative psychological evaluation of all surgical candidates in order to screen for psychopathology and prepare candidates for the many lifestyle changes expected after surgery. Bariatric surgery together with medical and behavioral followup is the most effective clinical approach to managing morbid obesity.[11]

A psychological evaluation is comprised of two main parts: the psychological testing and a clinical interview. With regard to psychological testing, the Minnesota Multiphasic Personality Inventory-2 is a frequently used instrument.[12] Although initially designed to be administered to psychiatric patients, it is used extensively with other categories of patients.

The clinical interview is comprised of a comprehensive assessment of the candidate's medical, surgical, and psychiatric history, drug or food allergies, history of eating disorders, alcohol or tobacco use, and both prescription and over-the-counter medications. The psychosocial history should also assess the candidate's family and social situation. Many times, family mem-

### UNDERSTANDING DEEP VEIN THROMBOSIS

Obesity increases the risk of deep vein thrombosis (DVT), a condition that disrupts the normal process of blood clotting. DVT occurs in approximately five percent of the population at some time in their lives, and this increases to 20 to 70 percent for hospitalized patients. DVT and subsequent pulmonary embolism (PE) are the leading causes of inpatient mortality in the US, leading to 200,000 deaths annually. DVT with PE poses the most serious threat to BWLS patients. DVT is characterized by thrombal occlusion of the deep veins of the leg. Homan's sign is the classic finding, although 50 percent of patients are asymptotic. Classic signs, often associated with other diagnosis, include cellulitis, hemoptysis, bruising or muscle strain. Patients might complain of shortness of breath, rapid pulse, excessive sweating, sharp pain, vertigo, or loss of consciousness. Doppler venous duplex ultrasound is a noninvasive diagnostic procedure that uses a transducer to determine the presence of a thrombus. It is the most common method of diagnosing DVT in the deep veins of the lower legs with 97 percent in the proximal vein, and 73 percent for calf vein. Venography is the most reliable method however, it is also the most invasive and expensive, and requires a high degree of expertise to read. Contrast medium is used in this uncomfortable procedure that occasionally leads to phlebitis. MRI is occasionally employed when diagnosis cannot be made with duplex venous ultrasound, or if the suspected embolus is elsewhere in the body.[16,17]

bers are also overweight, and this may be important for the patient's long-term success. The patient's knowledge of the surgery they are seeking should also be assessed. It is important to make certain that the patient has the evaluation far enough in advance of surgery that any preoperative recommendations can be well underway and not delay progress. For example, at the survey and the clinical interview, the results of the psychological tests are reviewed with the candidate. This is the time that additional questions and concerns are addressed. Any

preoperative recommendations are also made. Some programs require a written contract with the candidate and perhaps his/her support person. The written contract outlines any agreement, commitment, requirements or specific responsibilities necessary before surgery is scheduled.

### SURGICAL OPTIONS

From a historical perspective, bariatric weight loss surgery was first performed in the mid-twentieth century. This was largely due to the clinical observation that patients having the BillRoth II seemed to

**SAMPLE APPROVAL DOCUMENT**

**Bariatric Surgery Decision Support Tool**
**BlueCross BlueShield of Tennessee**

Patient Name: _____Age: ____Date: ___
Provider's name:_____
Provider's address: _____
Provider's phone number: _____
Diagnosis code(s): _____
CPT code(s): _____
Date Services are to be rendered: _____
Member's ID:_____

**Please provide the following documentation:**

**Name of specific bariatric surgical procedure:**
**Is the individual 18 years old or older?**
**Does the individual have a diagnosis of morbid obesity that has persisted for at least five years?**
**What is the individual's body mass index (BMI) and height / weight?**
- **Is the individual's BMI above 40 kg/m²? (List any applicable comorbidities)**
- **Is the individual's BMI equal to 35 kg/m²? List the obesity related comorbidities that will reduce the individual's life expectancy.**

**Does the individual have three (3) or more cardiac risk factors? Please list them.**
**What methods did the individual use to lose weight? (e.g., pharmacotherapy, Weight Watchers® low fat diets, exercise, lifestyle modification) Please provide the beginning and ending dates of each method attempted and failed.**
**Did the individual lose weight, gain weight, or stay the same during the weight loss attempts?**
**Or was the individual unable to comply with the requirements of the diet?**

**The documentation below must be submitted prior to authorization of the service:·**

- **Evidence that the attempt at conservative management was within two (2) years prior to the planned surgery.**
- **The attending physician (not the operating surgeon and his / her associates) must submit the documentation of the conservative management failures (this includes the information related to the methods used by the individual in the attempt to lose weight, including a nutritional consultation). Note: The bariatric surgeon requesting the surgical procedure can submit the information provided by the attending physician, with the authorization request.**
- **The attending physician must submit documentation that the individual can adhere to the pre and postoperative programs. This information should include, assessment of levels of depression, eating disorders, stress management, cognitive abilities, self esteem, and personality traits that may affect treatment, readiness and ability to adhere to the required lifestyle modifications and follow-up.·**
- **The attending physician who is managing the care and weight loss of the individual must submit a recommendation for the bariatric surgery due to the failure of conservative therapy. Note: The bariatric surgeon requesting the surgical procedure can submit the recommendation from the attending physician with the authorization request.[18]**

lose weight postoperatively. This sparked interest in a surgical approach to weight loss.[8]

Today, two main categories of surgery are used to treat morbid obesity. These are gastric restrictive and combined gastric restriction and malabsorption. With gastric restriction, the size and capacity of the stomach are limited. The stomach pouch is often reduced to 15 to 30 milliliters.

The Roux-en-Y Gastric Bypass (RYGB) combines gastric restriction and malabsorption and is the most common procedure done in the US today. This procedure creates a small pouch with an anastomosis to the jejunum. Food the patient eats bypasses 90 percent of the stomach and duodenum and a limb of jejunum in varying lengths and thus fewer calories are absorbed. When high caloric foods are dumped into the limb of the small intestine, a feeling of satiety or even discomfort may result, helping to curb the appetite.[9] Reduced consumption and/or absorption of the food leads to weight loss. This procedure can be done laparoscopically in certain patients.

In vertical banded gastroplasty, a vertical line of surgical staples is used to create the pouch, and a polypropylene band is placed at the lower end of the pouch. This band creates a stoma that won't stretch and provides for an outlet into the small intestine. With circumgastric banding, also restrictive, stomach size is limited by an inflatable band placed around the fundus of the stomach. The band is connected to a subcutaneous port and can be inflated or deflated in the provider's office. This is done to change the stoma size to meet the patient needs as he or she loses weight. Banding can be done laparoscopically, making it less invasive than stapling and a better choice for some categories of patients. In both procedures, patients need to follow the diet restrictions closely to avoid overstretching. Risks associated with the restrictive procedure include vomiting from overstretching the small pouch, band slippage or wearing away of the band, or leakage of stomach contents into the abdominal cavity. This method used alone has limited success in achieving long-term weight loss.

Malabsorptive surgery bypasses a length of small intestine. By bypassing a segment of the small intestine, weight loss occurs. This procedure can result in more weight loss than restrictive methods, and therefore is more effective in reducing comorbidities.

Malabsorptive procedures are less commonly used because of risks involved. Risks involved with malabsorptive procedures include liver disease, osteoporosis, diarrhea, dehydration, electrolyte imbalances, and malnutrition. Signs of malnutrition include but are not limited to: hair loss, anemia, edema, and vitamin depletion. Dumping syndrome, which is characterized by nausea, weakness, sweating, and diarrhea after certain meals and especially with concentrated sweets, occurs when the food moves too quickly out of the stomach and into the intestines.

Like RNYGB, the biliopancreatic diversions (BPD) are a combination procedure in that they both have a restrictive and a malabsorptive component. The BPD involves removing a portion of the stomach and creating a long limb Roux-en-Y connection. A reduction of oral intake and an increase in malabsorption occurs. Patients are able to eat larger quantities of food and still lose weight. Side effects of this procedure include flatus, loose and/or foul smelling stools, and stomal ulcers. As previously mentioned, malnutrition, especially protein malnutrition, can occur.

Adding a duodenal switch to the traditional BPD procedure results in a BPD/DS procedure. A portion of the stomach is removed, but the remaining stomach remains attached to the duodenum. The duodenum is then connected to the jejunum. The food then bypasses much of the small intestine resulting in fewer calories absorbed and subsequent weight loss. Complications are similar to the BPD procedure except that stomal ulceration and dumping syndrome are virtually eliminated.[13]

## MANAGING COMPLICATIONS

Assessment and documentation of vital signs are imperative, especially if a change in the clinical condition occurs. Pain management is a priority. This may be accomplished by giving pain medications via various routes. Non-narcotic implantable pain pumps can be used to decrease the pain at the incision site without the threat of an adverse respiratory consequence. Respiratory consequences such as postoperative atelectasis and pneumonia are common complications that can be minimized by early ambulation, repositioning, use of incentive spirometry, coughing, and deep breathing.

The patient may have a gastric tube; this should be monitored based strictly on the surgeon's expressed recommendations. All other tubes and catheter must be monitored for patency and fluid balance. All intake and output must be documented in the patient record, and output should include information on color, consistency, odor, and amount.

Deep venous thrombosis prevention is especially important among obese patients. Sequential compression devices and compression stockings must be size-appropriate.

The patient will have had instructions on postoperative nutrition, but a nutrition consult should occur to review diet needs and evaluate the patient's understanding of such.

## NUTRITIONAL CONSIDERATIONS

Most patients having BWLS are able to avoid nutritional problems if monitored properly. However, dehydration, protein malnutrition, and vitamin and mineral deficiencies may still occur. Mild dehydration can occur in the early postoperative period and is due to the decreased intake associated with limited gastric capacities. Vomiting and diarrhea both exacerbate fluid loss. Fluid balance is unique to each patient, and therefore patients are instructed to use thirst and urine concentration as a guide for fluid intake. Additionally, patients are instructed to consume approximately 60 to 80 grams of protein daily. If the patient is meat-intolerant, then protein supplements may be necessary. In the event of malabsorption, protein may be lost in the stool, and serum protein levels may help clinicians

determine the individual's protein requirements. Supplemental iron may be necessary for patients who are meat-intolerant. Most patients can be maintained with diet and a daily complete vitamin and calcium.

Recommendations suggest that patients take 325mg of an iron compound, 500 to 600mcg of $B_{12}$, 1mg of folate, and 500 to 1,000mg of calcium daily. In the malabsorptive procedures, more deficiencies can occur; therefore, fat-soluble vitamins, electrolytes such as sodium, potassium, chloride, phosphorous, magnesium, and zinc, and other vitamins and minerals should be monitored with serum levels. Patients with significant vomiting or poor food intake and women of child-bearing age may require additional assessment and supplementation.[14]

## LONG-TERM IMPLICATIONS OF BWLS

A patient will be required to have lifetime monitoring of weight, comorbidities, and nutritional status. The surgical procedure is considered to be a success if 50 percent of excess weight is lost and the patient maintains his/her weight loss for five years. Improvement or resolution of comorbidities is expected. This includes type 2 diabetes, sleep apnea, hypertension, infertility, depression, asthma, gastroesophageal reflux disease (GERD), back pain, and urinary incontinence. A patient who is planning to become pregnant should not do so for one year postoperatively or until her weight has stabilized. Rapid weight loss and nutritional deficiencies can harm a growing fetus.

For many postoperative bariatric surgery patients, food had become a coping mechanism and part of their support system. The change in lifestyle is dramatic and support groups are necessary to celebrate as well as cope with the loss. Long-term followup to discuss the physical, social, and psychosocial implications of the new lifestyle are the basis of success.

## *SUMMARY*

The number of obese people is increasing and, concurrently, surgical options are improving. Realistically, while some patients will do poorly, many are experiencing a dramatic improvement in quality of life with BWLS. The key to BWLS is an interdisciplinary team effort which is comprised of clinical experts, specially-designed equipment, and adequate resources.

## *REFERENCES*

1. Clinical guidelines on the identification, evaluation, and treatment of overweight and obesity in adults. *Obes Res* 1998;6:51s–209s.
2. Gallagher S. Taking the weight off with bariatric surgery. *Nursing* 2004;34(3):58–64.
3. Gastrointestinal Surgery for Severe Obesity. NIH Consensus Statement Online 1991;9(1):1–20.
4. Finklestrein E, Fiebelkorn I, Wang G. State-level estimates of annual medical expenditures attributable to obesity. *Obes Res* 2004;18–24.
5. Finklestrein E, Fiebelkorn I, Wang G. National medical expenditures attributable to overweight and obesity: How much and who's paying? *Health Affairs* 2003;3:219––26
6. Strum R. The effects of obesity, smoking, and drinking on medical conditions and cost. *Health Affairs* 2002;21:245–53.
7. Magee M. The cost of obesity in America. Available at: www.health-politics.com/program_transript.asp?p=prog_47. Access date: March 2005.
8. Buchwald H, Avidor Y, Braunwald E, et al. Bariatric surgery: A systematic review and meta-analysis. *J Am Med Assoc* 2004;292:1724–37.
9. Obesity Surgery Specialists. Benefits of surgery. Available at: www.obesity-surgery-center.com/benefits_gastric_bypass_surgery.htm. Access date: May, 2005.
10. Garza S. Bariatric weight loss surgery: Patient education, preparation, and follow-up. *Crit Care Nurs Q* 2003;26(2):101–4.
11. Buchwald H. Mainstreaming bariatric surgery. *Obes Surg* 1991;9:462–70.
12. MMPI- 2 The Minnesota Report. Regents of the University of Minnesota 2001.
13. Woodward B. Bariatric surgery options. *Crit Care Nurs Q* 2003;26(2):89–100.
14. Deitel M, Shikora SA. The development of surgical treatment of morbid obesity. *J Am Coll Nutr* 2002;21(5):365–71.
15. Cowan SM, Wallace RD, Marx A, Hiller ML. Plastic surgery after loss of massive excess weight. In: Deitel M, Cowan GSM (eds). *Update: Surgery for the Morbidly Obese Patient Toronto, Canada.* Toronto: FD-Communications, 2000.
16. All about DVT: Know the signs. Accessed at: www.dvt.net/signsSymptoms.do. Access date: May 2005.
17. Health effects of obesity. AOA Fact Sheet. American Obesity Association. Accessed at: www.obesity.org/education/health.shtml. Access date: May 2005.
17. Bariatric Surgery Decision Tree. Blue Cross Blue Shield of Tennessee. Accessed At: www.bcbst.com/MPManual/Bariatric_Surgery_Questionnaire.htm. Access date: May 2005.

# Medical Weight Loss

**4**

**O**besity is directly associated with a number of chronic conditions, many of which are physically and emotionally disabling. As the rate of obesity increases, so do concerns about individual and public health. Emotional and economic costs associated with obesity continue to climb. Typically people who participate in medical weight loss programs and lose 10 percent of their weight will regain almost all of it within five years. Obesity must be viewed as a chronic condition, with ongoing education, encourage-ment, and support. This chapter addresses the meaning of weight loss, barriers to change, traditional weight loss tools, and ways patients operationalize them. Case studies are included, along with resources and websources.

## THE MEANING OF WEIGHT LOSS

Diets as we understand them today consist of food and drink that we use to sustain the body. When the term *diet* is used, it usually is in conjunction with losing, gaining, or maintaining weight.

Many people are preoccupied with their physical appearance and with weight loss, and therefore dieting. Unrealistic expectations in terms of physical appearance lead to unrealistic notions about weight loss, and therein paves the way for fad or extreme diets and behaviors.

Several centuries ago, dieting focused more heavily on eating nutritious food in order to prevent or combat certain nutrition-related illness, and weight gain was admired as it provided a hedge against famine. As food became more readily available, people no longer needed to make such a concerted effort to incorporate certain nutrients into their diets. In fact, the opposite occurred, and somehow the trend was redirected toward a thinner body habitus. The ability to maintain a thinner body is more difficult than ever before in history, probably due to the abundance and delicious nature of high fat, calorie-dense foods coupled with the inability to get adequate physical activity. These factors lead to weight gain, which leads to feelings of desperation among many who cannot seem to control their body weight. The phenomenon of weight loss has taken on qualities consistent with those of cult-like behaviors,

## TABLE 1: CALCULATING BODY MASS INDEX

**B**ody mass index (BMI) can be used to measure both overweight and obesity in adults. BMI does not directly measure percent of body fat, but it provides a more accurate measure of overweight and obesity than relying on weight alone. BMI is found by dividing a person's weight by height in meters squared. See http://www.nhlbisupport.com/bmi for a BMI calculator. The mathematical formula is: weight(kg)/height squared (m²).

**NIDDK. Statistics related to overweight and obesity. Accessed at: www.niddk.nih.gov**

in that those participating in fad diets have feelings of overwhelming hopelessness and are looking at a way to literally transform themselves.[1] It becomes the clinician's responsibility to identify these behaviors and caution patients against claims promising "28 pounds and three pant sizes in two weeks" or "bikini body in 10 days—guaranteed."

## GOALS

Despite the well recognized need for weight control, patients, families, and clinicians are often disappointed in weight loss efforts. For example, weight loss based solely on decreasing intake has proved less than successful for most dieters. In fact, severely restrictive diets may lead to binge patterns, which further erode the patient's self esteem and ability to control weight.

Recent research suggests a more modest approach to weight loss. Previously it was thought that the goal of weight loss activities was to achieve ideal body weight or close to it. Today, however, if improving health is the aim, the goal is a 5 to 15 percent weight loss.

## UNDERSTANDING READINESS

What patients learn, how they learn, and how much they learn depends on many factors. Among the most important factors are the patient's physical and emotional well being. Unfortunately, many lifestyle changes must begin when the patient has little physical or emotional reserves--perhaps after a long and exhaustive hospitalization. The clinician's goal is two-fold in this instance, and the first is to find the method that most fully supports the patient's support system, meaning family or friends that care for the patient. The second is to

## BARRIERS TO MAKING CHANGES

**P**rimary care providers are encouraged to play a more active role in making recommendations to patients who are categorically described as obese. Several expert panels have developed algorithms for the assessment and treatment of weight issues. The challenge this poses, then, is how primary providers ought to introduce these lifestyle changes to the patient, and what vocabulary ought to be used in discussions with patients. Patients are often offended by terms such as obese and fat, yet others might be offended by euphemisms…responding with, "I'm fat, look at me, I'm comfortable with my body…why aren't you?"

For more on algorithms and how best to address patients, see:
1. Galuska DA, Will JC, Serdula MK, Ford ES. Are healthcare professionals advising patients to lose weight. *J Am Med Assoc* 1999;282:1576-8.
2. Guidance for Treatment of adult Obesity. Available at: shapeup.org.
3. Wadden TA, Anderson KA, Foster GD, et al. Obese women's perception of their physicians' weight management attitudes and practices. *Arch Fam Med* 2000;9:854–60.
4. Wadden TA, Didie E. What's in a name? Patients' preferred terms for describing obesity. *Obes Research* 2003:11:1140–6.

help the healthcare organization and other disciplines to be responsive to the wide range of development levels, backgrounds, experiences, and needs that patients bring with them.

Patients must drive the weight loss process. The term readiness, by definition, means that the patient has expressed interest in weight loss, understands that weight management is a lifelong commitment, and is able to take the appropriate steps to make necessary lifestyle changes.

## THEORIES

Weight loss is achieved by mobilizing the body's fat stores, and can only be accomplished when an energy deficit exists. A number of both widely publicized and little known methods are used to create this energy deficit. Regardless, simply stated, obesity occurs when input (calories in) exceeds output (activity expended).[2] The reverse is true for weight loss. Despite the countless theories to explain weight regulation, in order for a decrease in weight to occur, activity expended must exceed calories consumed.

## DIETARY CONSIDERATIONS

Any time calorie consumption is decreased, it becomes important to address nutrition and the nutritional requirements of the individual. The patient must receive training in healthy eating such as selecting lower fat foods, increasing quality proteins, and increasing fruits, vegetables, and grains. Individually planned diets usually create a deficit of 500 to 1,000 calories per day and are aimed at a weight loss of one to two pounds per week. Physician-supervised weight loss programs might include a very low calorie diet (VLCD), and vitamin and nutritional supplements, together with exercise and lifestyle changes, to bring about a rapid weight loss. The VLCD should only be used under the careful supervision and monitoring of a physician or other specially trained healthcare clinician.[3] While most weight loss takes place because of decreased calorie intake, sustained physical activity is necessary to provide a healthier lifestyle and a long-term outcome.

## EXERCISE

The primary manner of increasing energy expenditure is through physical activity. When the person is ready for weight loss, it is important to incorporate activity, as exercise is more successful in lowering the risk of cardiovascular disease and diabetes than just weight loss alone.

## THREAT OF FAT

I have spent years dieting, and I have tried hundreds of diets--the grapefruit diet, cabbage soup diet, Russian Air Force Diet, Caveman diet, cellophane wraps, and I have even had my jaw wired. I didn't want to become a better me...I wanted to become a new me. I never thought about it as a cult behavior, but if I understand this correctly, the dietitian explained that people are vulnerable to joining cults when they feel completely powerless or hopeless over their existence, and they want to be a completely transformed person. This is exactly what I have always tried to accomplish. It wasn't until she explained that I had a vulnerability to irresponsible fad diets because of my way of thinking that I began to understand how I was sabotaging my life. She spent a lot of time talking about responsible options for weight loss, but more importantly we both learned that without some level of counseling I would probably continue to sabotage my efforts. As cliché as it sounds, I needed to learn to care for me...to love me...to accept me. For more information on the size and weight advocacy groups, visit: naafa.org and cswd.org.

## FEAR OF THIN

Anna believes that her dilemma is probably similar to many other people who weight cycle or yo-yo diet. She explains that she is not comfortable when her body is thinner. She feels better physically, but fails to adjust emotionally. Anna is correct in her assessment that this is not an uncommon phenomenon. Clinicians must be prepared to address this obstacle to change. Barbara Thompson describes some of the issues that emerge with weight loss, such as spousal jealousy, dealing with new attention, divorce, friends' attitudes, and others. For more on the challenges of adapting to a new body, read: Thompson B. *Weight Loss Surgery: Finding the Thin Person Hiding Inside You!* Tarentum, PA: Word Association Publishers, 2002.

Additionally, studies suggest that physical activity will improve the long-term results of weight loss treatment, preserve lean body mass, and improve emotional well being and self esteem.

Options for physical activity range from simply taking advantage of everyday activities to enrolling in a formal fitness program. The intensity, duration, frequency, and type of physical activity will depend on the presence of any comorbidities, previous activity, and individual preferences. Experts agree that initially inactive individuals should begin by simply increasing opportunities to walk short distances, take the stairs when possible, etc. The challenge to heavier individuals is finding activities that accommodate weight and size. Additionally, some obese people avoid outdoor activities because of embarrassment.

Walking had gained increasing interest in the past few years, as more research is available to affirm its benefits. Still, some people are reluctant to engage in walking activities. In fact, a recent study from Ohio State University suggested that concern about neighborhood dangers was the primary reason women avoid walking for fitness. Clinicians serve patients by acknowledging this barrier and then discussing ideas for overcoming these concerns. Walkers should drive by a planned route at the time of day they believe they will be exercising, looking for dimly lit areas, unrestrained pets, unreasonable traffic, and other hazards. Consider carrying a can of pepper spray, which stops a dog or person without the threat of permanent injury. Encourage patients to find others who will walk with them, as there is safety in numbers.

Extreme climates pose other very realistic obstacles to walking. Whether the lem is long, freezing winters or hot, humid summers, patients will need ideas to overcome these issues. The first idea that comes to mind is walking the mall; many people prefer this because there are usually security guards, climate control, and other walkers! Others purchase gym equipment for home use, but keep in mind there may be weight limits to some equipment. Advise patients that perhaps other activities may be more appropriate in extreme climates; however, the most valuable advice is that once a patient breaks the exercise habit, it can become very difficult to start again. As a clinician, look to your own community to find resources for your larger patients—perhaps an indoor pool, a gym tailored to the needs of larger people, or other resources are available.

## DRUGS

Drug therapy may be considered for use among patients with a BMI of 30 or more without comorbidities, or 27 or more with comorbidities. Pharmaceutical intervention used as a treatment for obesity has historically failed to sustain long-term success. For example, consider amphetamines or the fen-phen combination, both producing serious side effects and ultimately being discontinued.

Just as there are some side effects for almost any type of drug, there are also side effects of obesity-related drugs. Some common side effects of appetite suppressants include dry mouth, dizziness, abdominal pain, diarrhea/constipation, nausea, difficulty sleeping, nervousness, hypertension, and headaches. While appetite suppressants generally suppress appetite, they may also alter the way the body burns calories. Among the most widely recognized categories of weight loss drugs are the amphetamines (amphetamine, dextroamphetamine, methamphetamine). Amphetamines are strong stimulants that are no

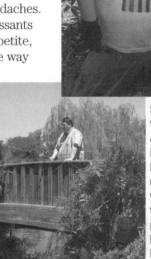

**Studies suggest that physical activity will improve the long-term results of weight loss treatment, preserve lean body mass, and improve emotional well being and self esteem.**

### FIT AND FAT

Today, more and more people are beginning to see medical charts as unscientific, impersonal, and even dangerous. David Alexander is in peak condition. He is 5'8" tall, and weighs 250 pounds—100 pounds more than the recommended weight for someone his height. However, David's physician says: David is fit! In a typical week, David swims five miles, runs 30 miles, and cycles 200 miles. He has completed 264 triathalons. David's resting pulse rate is in the 60s, and his blood pressure is usually in the 120s over 80s. The message to clinicians is that weight loss goals may differ from patient to patient and perhaps it is possible to be fit and fat! For more stories and to see the full interview with David Alexander, visit: pbs.org for Frontline 1708 "FAT" Aired November 3, 1998.

longer recommended by most authorities because they are highly addictive and lead to numerous side effects. Side effects include heart palpitations, hypertension, gastrointestinal disturbances, and insomnia. However, recently several newer drugs have been introduced, and in certain patients, pharmaceutical therapy can augment the effects of a plan comprised of nutrition, activity, and behavioral therapy.

Several weight loss drugs recently introduced are thought to be promising thus far. To reinforce, drugs are never a substitute for lifestyle changes, and therefore drug treatment should be used in combination with a healthy diet, physical activity, and behavioral therapy. Regular follow-up visits to the primary care provider are recommended to monitor progress, and to reinforce/reevaluate and maintain safety of the drug's use.

Weight loss drugs approved by the US Food and Drug Administration (FDA) for treating obesity include Orlistat, Sibutramine, and Phentermine. Sibutramine (Meridia, Abbott Laboratories) and Orlistat (Xenical, Hoffman-LaRoche) are two drugs indicated for long-term use. Long-term drugs are typically associated

---

**FIRST PERSON**

I have lost almost 1,200 pounds in the past five years...not all at one time, though. What I am trying to say is that I yo-yo. I give up everything in my life to lose weight, which I can do. But, unfortunately, the weight finds me once I get back to a normal life. Today, and in the past 15 months, I have maintained a weigh of 162 pounds and I feel great. My body and my spirit are healthy. You might ask, "What made the difference"? Well, let me share: I visited Martha, the nurse practitioner at my OB-GYN's office almost two years ago. Instead of giving me a diet and activity plan, she actually talked to me for about an hour. We talked about my previous attempts at permanent weight loss. She said that she felt the issue was not my ability to lose weight, but my ability to adapt the unrealistic sequestered lifestyle wherein I lose weight to a more practical real lifestyle. I had to agree. She gave me some factors to consider in developing long-term success at weight loss. These were a few of the issues she wanted me to consider:

• Is the program I chose convenient to my home and work?
• Do I have safe and reliable transportation to travel to the program of choice?
• Do I have enough disposable financial resources to pay for my program of choice?
• Do I have enough time to allow for follow-through?

Martha was exactly right. The last time I lost weight I had joined a weight training program at the local college, which was so much fun, but when the time changed and it got darker earlier, I just didn't feel safe there any longer. I was uncomfortable in the general parking lot and couldn't afford the close lot. I couldn't leave work earlier to take advantage of the daylight hours—it was a problem all the way around. These were huge barriers that I didn't anticipate. I sabotaged my own efforts without even thinking!

---

with a 5 to 10 percent weight loss that is sustained for one year when used with in conjunction with diet and activity. Sibutramine, which works as an appetite suppressant, became available in February 1997 for long-term use.

Orlistat first became available in the US in May 1999. It is not an appetite suppressant, but rather a lipase inhibitor, and works by blocking about 30 percent of

dietary fat from being absorbed.[4] It is meant to work along with a low-calorie, low-fat diet. Some side effects include oily spotting, flatulence with discharge, fecal urgency, oily evacuation, and fecal incontinence. Additionally, Orlistat interferes with fat-soluble vitamin absorption. Maintaining a diet consisting of less than 30-percent fat calories may minimize these side effects.

**THE TWELVE STEPS OF OVEREATERS ANONYMOUS**

1. **We admitted we were powerless over food—that our lives had become unmanageable.**
2. **Came to believe that a Power greater than ourselves could restore us to sanity.**
3. **Made a decision to turn our will and our lives over to the care of God as we understood Him.**
4. **Made a searching and fearless moral inventory of ourselves.**
5. **Admitted to God, to ourselves, and to another human being the exact nature of our wrongs.**
6. **Were entirely ready to have God remove all these defects of character.**
7. **Humbly asked Him to remove our shortcomings.**
8. **Made a list of all persons we had harmed and became willing to make amends to them all.**
9. **Made direct amends to such people wherever possible, except when to do so would injure them or others.**
10. **Continued to take personal inventory and when we were wrong, promptly admitted it.**
11. **Sought through prayer and meditation to improve our conscious contact with God as we understood Him, praying only for knowledge of His will for us and the power to carry that out.**
12. **Having had a spiritual awakening as the result of these Steps, we tried to carry this message to compulsive overeaters and to practice these principles in all of our affairs.**

*Permission to use the Twelve Steps of Alcoholics Anonymous for adaptation granted by AA World Services, Inc.*

Patients are advised to take a daily supplement that contains vitamins A, D, E, K, and beta-carotene.[5]

Phentermine is an appetite suppressant that was first approved by the FDA in 1959 as a short term adjunct in a regimen of weight reduction based on caloric restriction. It is sold under the brand names Lonamin, Adipex, Fastin, Banobese, Obenix, and Zantryl. Phentermine, which remains in use, is half of the combination therapy fen-phen. The use of phen-termine alone has not been associated with the adverse health risks of the fenflu-ramine-phentermine combination.[6]

## SURGERY

The concept of gastrointestinal surgery to control obesity grew out of weight loss that resulted from operations for cancer or severe ulcers that removed a part of the stomach or small intestine. The surgery promotes weight loss by restricting food intake, and in some ver-sions, interrupting digestive processes. In 2004, almost 144,000 surgeries were performed. The challenge to patients is that today most surgeons need the patient to lose some weight before surgery. This becomes necessary because with the overall weight loss, the abdominal organs also will become smaller, and this creates an added advantage during the surgical procedure. Additionally, patients and clinicians who fully understand medical weight loss strategies can be of help to patients struggling to lose weight after surgery.

## INDIVIDUAL

Although most individuals prefer some level of support, some patients prefer to engage in self-help weight loss. Any effort that patients make to lose weight themselves qualifies as self help. The patient can either purchase, download, or borrow weight loss materials and use them at home. Patients losing weight at home through use of self-help resources could fall prey to fad or extreme behaviors. Encourage patients to seek support if they feel overwhelmed by this approach.

## COMMUNITY

Sometimes referred to as non-clinical, non-commercial

programs, community-based weight loss programs are provided one-on-one, in groups, or as a combination. TOPS (Taking Off Pounds Sensibly) and OA (Overeaters Anonymous) are two such examples.

TOPS is a non-profit support group system that has served overweight people for over 50 years. TOPS does not have their own diet; instead, motivation and support are the focus. Although no claims have been made as to the safety or success of this program, groups support and weekly weigh-ins can be very helpful to participants.[7]

Overeaters Anonymous is more structured than TOPS. The Twelve Steps are the heart of the OA recovery program, offering a new way of life that enables the compulsive eater to live without the need for excessive food. The ideas expressed in the Twelve Steps, which originated in Alcoholics Anonymous, reflect practical experience and application of spiritual insights recorded by thinkers throughout the ages.[8] The common thread in these programs is mutual support and encouragement.

## INDUSTRY

Formal commercial programs include Diet Workshop, Richard Simmons, Weight Watchers, Curves, and

## WHOSE WEIGHT IS IT?

My father constantly talks about my weight—not just to me, but to everyone. I haven't seen him for almost a year because of his behavior. Since the last time I saw him I have made two positive life changes. The first is to commit to one bowl of Cheerios and two pieces of fruit before 2 o'clock in the afternoon. I know that sounds silly, but if I eat these foods in that time framework, I control feelings of guilt and I have fewer cravings...I don't know why, but it works for me. Anyway, I have lowered my cholesterol and lost 17 pounds in 12 months. The second positive change is to walk one mile three days a week. I really think this controls stress. I am becoming stronger each day, and was just about to embark on a more rigorous life of more activity and better nutrition when I learned I was pregnant. I will still eat properly and do lots of activity, but I am aware there are times when a person should not try to lose weight. The temporary exclusions for weight loss are pregnancy, lactation, unstable mental illness, and unstable physical condition. Exclusions that require clinical judgment include osteoporosis and cholelithiasis. Those that constitute permanent exclusion are anorexia nervosa and terminal illness. I am simply pregnant and look forward to more aggressive weight loss efforts once the baby is weaned. In the meantime, I have found several websites that offer very cute maternity wear for larger women. I may be heavier than most mothers, but I am strong and healthy and I am going to be a beautiful, happy, pregnant mother-to-be. My father may not see me that way, but I do!

Maternity resource:
• www.radiancemagazine.com/marketplace
• www.plus-size-pregnancy.org

More reading on walking:
• Aerobic Walking The Weight Loss Exercise: A Complete Guide to Reduce Weight, Stress, and Hypertension by Mort Malkin
• Be Alert, Be Aware, Have a Plan by Neal Rawls
• Fitness for Dummies by Suzanne Schlosberg
• Fitness Walking by Therese Iknoian
• Fitness Walking for Dummies by Liz Neporent
• The Spirited Walker: Walking for Clarity, Balance, and Spiritual Connection by Carolyn S. Kortge
• The 90-Day Fitness Walking Program by Mark Fenton
• Walking Fast by Therese Iknoian
• Walking Handbook by Susan B. Johnson
• Walking Magazine Complete Guide to Walking: For Health, Fitness, and Weight Loss by Mark Fenton

Websources for fitness walking:
www.WalkBlaster.com
www.powerbelt.com
www.fitnessjournal.org

**LIFESTYLE CHANGES**
- **Keep a diary to record eating and activity patterns**
- **Learn new stress management skills**
- **Identify self-defeating environmental cues**
- **Self-reward for positive behaviors**
- **Rethink goals of health and weight**

Jenny Craig. These highly structured programs are of consistent quality, outcomes, and philosophy, regardless of geographic locations. Some are more costly than others. Clinicians should be aware of the industry-based services in their community in order to make responsible choices available to patients.

## MEDICALLY SUPERVISED

Direct patient involvement with a physician, nurse expert (such as a nurse practitioner, or clinical nurse specialist), registered dietitian, exercise physiologist, social worker, clinical psychologist, counselor or other weight loss specialist constitutes a medically-supervised weight loss program. Research suggests that this category of weight loss program yields the best short- and long-term success. Some hospitals are developing Wellness Centers that are clinician-driven options for patients. Other examples of medically supervised weight loss programs

include: Medifast, Optifast, Healthy Solutions, and New Directions. Medically supervised programs usually are well documented in terms of clinical outcomes. For example, Medifast alone has been available for over 20 years, and used by over a million patients.

## CONCLUSION

In summary, a comprehensive medical weight loss program should consist of patient assessment to include medical history, physical examination, and lab and diagnostic studies such as an electrocardiogram to ensure the patient is a candidate for weight loss. A mutual understanding of patient readiness, resources, and support should be addressed before weight loss efforts are introduced. Appropriate instruction should include nutrition, activity, lifestyle changes, and medications based on patient needs.

Consider diet and nutrition, including a reduced calorie diet or VLCD and dietary supplement as needed. Safe, effective activity that is tailored to the ability, preferences, resources, and limitations of the patient should be discussed. Lifestyle changes must be discussed in order to include an understanding of proper nutrition, stress, family, and good health in general. Consider prescription appetite suppression and other avail-

able medications if indicated in a comprehensive medical weight loss program. Recognize that each person is unique and their manner of implementing change will be unique, whether the patient prefers a group setting, clinically supervised setting, or opts to use a more individualized strategy. The role of the clinician is to stay informed on the latest development in weight loss and health promotion, and to support and encourage the patient.

## REFERENCES

1. Hoffer E. *The True Believer: Thoughts on the Nature of Mass Movements.* New York: Harper and Row, 1951.
2. National Institutes of Health. Clinical guidelines on the identification, evaluation, and Treatment of overweight and obesity in adults. *Obes Res* 1998;6:51s–209s.
3. What are some medical weight loss tips? American Society of Bariatric Physicians. Available at: www.asbp.org/faq.htm#7. Access date: May 2005.
4. Kromer J, Arrone LJ. Pharmaceutical approaches to weight reduction: Therapeutic targets. *J Clin Endocrinol Metabol* 2004;89(6):2616–21.
5. What are the different categories of diet medications? American Society of Bariatric Physicians. Available at: www.asbp.org/faq.htm#9. Access date: May 2005.
6. Drug Therapy. American Obesity Association Available at: www.obesity.org/treatment/weight.shtml. Access date: May 2005.
7. What is TOPS? Available at: www.icomm.ca/bctops/why.html. Access date: May 2005.
8. Overeaters Anonymous. The Twelve Steps. Accessed at: http://www.oa.org. Access date: May 2005.

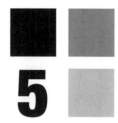

**5**

# Learning Theory

Obesity can seldom be cured and instead should be managed much the same way as any other chronic illness. Although a number of prevention, treatment, and maintenance strategies exist, the underlying goal is to provide clinical intervention that ensures long-term support, education, monitoring, and reinforcement. Specially trained clinical staff, comprised of dietitians, counselors, nurses, physicians, and others are in an excellent position to recognize and intervene with patients who are at risk and who could benefit from health-promoting activities. Making lifelong behavioral changes is difficult for everyone, but especially for individuals who have had long-term failure in managing a complex chronic condition such as obesity.

Understanding the challenges inherent in learning new behaviors and changing old behaviors can be overwhelming for patients, their families/friends, and their clinicians. This chapter argues for inclusion of clinicians in the

**INFORMED REFUSAL**

The aim of medical records and documentation therein is to tell a story about what has transpired between the clinician and the patient in a clear, consistent, complete, objective, timely manner. It has been increasingly important to include evidence of discussions concerning informed consent as well as informed refusal. As healthcare more fully embraces respect for personal autonomy, many patients are asserting their right to refuse treatment. What is the expectation when a 470-pound, 25-year-old patient refuses simple diagnostic tests in the primary care office, such as blood pressure readings? This situation requires active listening and discussion. It is increasingly recognized that clinicians have a responsibility to present factual information pertaining to the consequences inherent in refusing certain types of clinical intervention. If the patient continues to refuse after a thorough and responsible discussion, then the savvy clinician ought to consider informed refusal. Some contend the purpose of informed refusal is to prevent the risk of legal claim, but others feel that, like behavioral contracts, the document very specifically outlines the proposed treatment/intervention, explanation of risks and benefits, and consequences in refusal. A signed copy should be provided to the patient.

To read more, please see:
Nisonson I. Update your record-keeping skills: Informed consent and refusal. *Bull Am Coll Surgeons* 2000;85(5):18–22.

process and describes several ways to consider learning and changing.

## UNDERSTANDING THE POWER TO CHANGE

From birth, our behavior is aimed at doing what we believe will best satisfy one or more of our needs. At an early age human beings can tell the difference between pain and pleasure, and newborn babies quickly learn to express themselves so that those who take care of them can tell whether they are feeling good or bad. Parents may not know exactly how to help the baby feel better, but they almost always know how the baby feels. Very quickly babies learn to express when something is wrong, and parents learn to respond to that emotion. By using information around them, babies learn what feels good and what feels bad, and how to satisfy their needs by obtaining what they need from others around them.[1]

Even before starting school, most preschoolers are told by their families that they can expect to feel good in school; and initially it does feel good to be in school. But most agree that something changes; school, or the inherent hard work associated with it, no longer feels good. By junior high school, most children fail to find the fun in school, even though they are reminded that the sacrifice today will help them feel good later. For many children, school no longer satisfies their needs. Instead, human beings spend the rest of their lives trying to learn how to satisfy these needs, but most people do not have a clear idea of what these needs really are.

By the time overweight patients arrive in healthcare clinics and hospitals, many have tried every diet and exercise plan known to man. Like the junior high school student who has become disillusioned with school, so the obese person is disillusioned with weight loss plans. Patients are reminded by clinicians to continue working hard now, but also be patient because there will be less that feels good immediately, and more that will not feel good until later. The problem is that the genetic needs themselves know nothing about the concept of "later," and they are continuing to compel us to do what feels good now. In the case of diet-induced hunger, the dieter can tell his stomach to tolerate the discomfort of today's hunger in exchange for feeling better about himself later when weight loss ensues. But the man's stomach will not stop telling him that he needs food to satisfy one of the basic human needs. The longer the man diets, the more powerfully his stomach responds. This serves to begin the conflict dieters face everyday—this basic human drives results in feelings of personal failure.

Some clinicians believe if they could just do a better job of motivating the patient, the weight loss process would prove more successful for all involved. However, Glasser[2] explains that motivation as a commonly used word is largely misunderstood. Motivation must come from within, and it is impossible to "motivate" another person. Clinicians and patients only possess the power to motivate, or more accurately, to control *themselves*. By saying, "My patient lacks motivation," clinicians are more likely expressing, "I am frustrated because I lack the power to control the patient." As clinicians, we often try to control the behaviors of ourselves and others when, in fact, we can only control ourselves. Control theory gives permission to clinicians to stop controlling and become collaborative. The clinician's pater-

nalistic responsibility is transformed into a mutually responsive mentor:client relationship.

This is especially difficult for clinicians because of their professional commitment to health and outcome-based healthcare. All clinicians have experienced the angst of a suffering patient. Clinicians are in the position to see that if patients had avoided certain health-defeating activities throughout their lives, it's possible the suffering could have been avoided. This is the context that clinicians bring to the patient education encounter. This is why clinicians often behave paternalistically, because they have had experiences their patients don't fully under-

stand. However, an effective mentor provides sound information and realistic support that allows the client to take control of decision-making. This applies to all areas of chronic illness and other chronic conditions, including obesity.

Clinicians who are interested in working with their larger clients in addressing issues of health promotion best serve the client when they understand what drives the individual to engage in or resist change. Glasser reminds readers that both punishment and rewards are coercive and will create behavior change. However, he cautions that these changes are usually short-term.[2] Losing weight is difficult because the body is

## READINESS

I am so sick of hearing the phrases "readiness to learn" or "assessing readiness." I hate it when clinicians "clinicalize" my very personal experience. They produce a form that I complete or they begin asking the same questions I have been asked my whole life… "Why do you seek weight loss? Have you attempted weight loss before? With what degree of success?" No one asked me how they can help me reach my goals, I have never been addressed with any degree of respect. The questions are lifeless, without meaning or compassion. By the time I get to the clinic to ask for help with weight, I have been completely "beat up" in the public sphere. I want clinicians to support and encourage me when I am doing well, and respect how difficult all of this is when I fail. I may simply be your "9 o'clock appointment" but you are everything to me…by the time I make an appointment to see you, I have thought about you for months. Please just talk to me, care for me and about me, and help me learn to do the right things.

fighting the effort. This is an important consideration in healthcare.

Some clinicians and consumer groups remind healthcare providers that in most cases, health promotion activities will achieve greater success than a strict weight loss program only. Glasser might agree.

## ASSESSING READINESS

Clinicians must recognize their own readiness to mentor and support patients even before patient assessment. C. Everett Koop, the chairman and founder of *ShapeUp America!*, suggests clinicians examine their own feelings about obesity and the obese patient. Clinicians may harbor negative feelings that could influence the therapeutic relationship. Each patient must be viewed as a unique and competent individual worthy of time and respect. Clinicians must learn how the patient's obesity has affected his or her life and understand the factors that have contributed to weight gain. Encourage patients to discuss feelings about weight, weight loss, and weight maintenance efforts. Patients need to feel assured that clinicians are listening as they share their misconceptions, concerns, and frustrations. Weight loss choices

### USING CONTRACTS

**A**s clinicians, we believe that if we have done a good job teaching the patient, the patients will follow our recommendations...notice how clinician-driven this vocabulary feels. The patient isn't really part of the statement. Studies and clinical experience suggest that patients must be involved in the development and execution of all behavioral change affecting them and their lifestyles. One way to do this is to incorporate behavioral contracts, which specifically detail expectations, responsibilities, and actions of both the patient and clinician. Some experts believe contracts work because they tend to better clarify stakeholders' roles. Responsibility for attaining a goal transfers from the clinician to the patient. Contracts have been increasingly successful among obese patients requiring lifelong behavioral changes. Initially, patients must have a mutually responsive relationship with the clinician. Once a rapport has been established, the clinician can describe the rationale for the contract, including techniques for developing the contract and how priorities are established. Written contracts should be provided, and a signed copy should be kept by the patient. A good behavioral contract should consider the following:

- Clear, measurable overall goal
- Specific steps needed to reach overall goal
- Detailed time frame for initiation, evaluation, and modification
- Consequences if steps are not accomplished

Patients, families, friends, and clinicians have found that contracts are helpful in meeting the specific health promoting activities needed not only to survive, but thrive in the presence of chronic illness.

For more information on contracts, please visit:
Cosentino BW. I will, I will: Using contracts to promote positive patient behaviors. *Nursing Spectrum.* Available at: community.nursingspectrum.com/MagazineArticles/articles.cfm?AID=911. Access date: April, 2000.

and efforts must involve the patients and their family/friends. Decisions about treatments must be in partnership, patients must feel the therapeutic relationship is mutually responsive. Every effort must be made to recognize and comment

on positive changes in health-promoting behaviors such as change in health status, prevention of weight gain, weight loss, nutrition, activity, and overcoming individual barriers to change. Koop reminds clinicians that striving to forge a supportive

**ARTICLE REVIEWS**

**HOW DO PEOPLE PROCESS HEALTH INFORMATION? APPLICATIONS IN AN AGE OF INDIVIDUALIZED COMMUNICATION. Kreuter MW, Holt CL. *Current Directions in Psychological Science.* 2001;10(6):206–9.**

**SYNOPSIS: Studies suggest health education materials that are customized to the unique needs of the individual are more effective than generic handouts in eliciting behavioral changes. Advances in computer technology have made it possible to clinicians to individualize patient education materials. This article presents current research on methods patients use to process information, how this can be used today in patient care, and takes a look to the future.**

**ANTICIPATED EMOTIONS AS GUIDES TO CHOICE. Mellers BA. *Current Directions in Psychological Science.* 2001;10(6):210–14.**

**SYNOPSIS: The anticipation of emotion is likely to drive decisions that human beings make in all areas of life. Although this article does not address obesity specifically, it does offer a theory of anticipated pleasure that explains how life decisions are made, and how subjective the experience of pleasure actually is.**

relationship with each unique overweight patient throughout the change process ensures treatment that guarantees dignity and respect, which is essential to health promotion.[3]

Ultimately, Glasser would remind us, the decision to make life changes rests with the patient. Readiness means that the patient is interested in weight loss, understands the long-term commitment to change, and is willing to change behaviors to meet these goals. It is important to assess readiness as this determines the patient's medical, physical, and psychological ability to begin making changes. Clinicians must recognize that even if weight reduction is needed to reduce health risks, lack of readiness will negatively impact both long and short-term success.[4]

## FACTORS IN ASSESSING READINESS

The first indication that the patient is ready to learn new behaviors is the patient's expression to that extent. The patient should state the desire to make changes. Most patients will explain that they have engaged in weight loss efforts in the past, and clinicians should determine if this is the case. If so, how is the motivation at this time as compared to the past? Find out if there are conditions in the individual's personal life that might interfere with making changes. Determine if the patient gives the impression that he or she is ready to make a long-term commitment to change. Ask the patient to explain to what extent the obesity interferes with normal activities of daily living. For instance, is it comfortable and safe to drive a car? Does the seat belt fit safely and properly? Can the individual quickly and easily exit the car in case of emergency? Has there been employment or educational opportunities that were denied due to body weight?[5] Each of these factors helps clinicians understand better ways to begin the mentoring process, and help patients and their families/friends understand their ability to participate in new learned behaviors.

## POWERLESSNESS AND HEALTH-DEFEATING BEHAVIOR

Failure on the part of the patient to engage in health-promoting activities continues to perplex clinicians. It is a known fact that 60 percent of patients take their medications incorrectly, patients miss appointments, they may not follow through with treatments, and many times require an avoidable hospitalization directly related to health-defeating behaviors. Clinicians often misinterpret this behavior as resulting from issues such as basic lack of intelligence, convenience, cost, side effects, or one's value system. Others contend powerlessness is a factor in health-defeating behavior. If that is the case, the key to understanding patient behavior and changing the clinical approach is recognizing powerlessness.[6] Individuals who repeatedly fail to make strides over marginalized conditions may develop feelings of powerlessness. This is the case with some, but not all, obese patients.

Repeated failure at unreasonable weight loss regimens creates a climate of failure. Weight cycling, fad diets, and unrealistic goals all set the patient up for these negative emotions, and once firmly established within the essence of the person, self-esteem and hopefulness become eroded. Some individuals find relief from these feelings of powerlessness by using religion, ritual, or transcendent experiences to regain power over an otherwise hopeless situation. Others use a strategy described as "cope and defy." This individual typically rebels against the values

and traditions of the dominant or mainstream group. In the healthcare setting, that is usually characterized by rebelling against diet and exercise as presented in the form of handouts or brochures. Patients may openly challenge health-related theory, and this behavior is especially disturbing to the clinician whose value system is grounded in this theory. Lastly, substance abuse offers some patients a temporary transcendence over their otherwise hopeless condition. Religious transcendence, cope and defy, and substance abuse are all behaviors that help the person to feel better in the face of overwhelming adversity. The first message to clinicians is to work to prevent patients from feeling overwhelmed…health promoting behaviors do not always require weight loss. Behaviors such as proper footwear, healthier eating, and incremental increases in activity are all specific activities that are likely to be manageable and lead to a more positive lifestyle.

Paternalism is described as a dominant attitude of mainstream society over those who consider themselves marginalized. When paternalism exists in healthcare, the clinician cares for

the patient as a parent would care for a child. In paternalism, the ethical ideals of respect for personal autonomy and beneficence are in conflict because clinicians strive to do what is best for the patients (beneficence), at the risk of threatening respect for one's personal autonomy.

A paternalistic approach is not uncommon when clinicians care for those with chronic conditions such as obesity.[7] In order to avoid powerlessness and encourage a mutually responsive relationship, it is important that clinicians are aware of paternalism and the threat it poses to the therapeutic relationship.

## CONCLUSION

Most patients acknowledge repeated failure with weight loss regimens. These disappointments threaten meaningful change. Clinicians best serve overweight patients when they truly use evidence-based strategies to determine what is appropriate information to provide to the patient. Regardless, patients should be encouraged to avoid fad diets, unrealistic goals, and other meaningless methods of promoting a healthier lifestyle. The role of the clinician is to recognize the emotional and physical challenges necessary to make long-term changes in the face of a chronic condition and to work with each patient as a unique individual in a mutually responsive relationship.

## REFERENCES

1.  Glasser W. *Choice Theory: A New Psychology of Personal Freedom.* New York: HarperCollinsPublishers, 1998.
2.  Glasser W. *Control Theory: A New Explanation of How We Control Our Lives.* New York: Harper and Row, 1985.
3.  *Guidance for Treatment of Adult Obesity.* Available at: www.shapeup.org. Access date: May 2005.
4.  Robinson BE, Gjerdingen DK, Houge DR. Obesity: A move from traditional to more patient-oriented management. *J Am Board Fam Pract* 1995;355-63.
5.  Brownell K. *The LEARN Program for Weight Management.* Dallas, TX: American Publishing Company, 2000.
6.  Gallagher SM. Powerlessness as a factor in health defeating behavior. *Ost Wound Manage* 1997;43:34–42.
7.  Gallagher SM. The meaning of otherness in health care planning. *Ost Wound Manage* 1999;45:16–18.

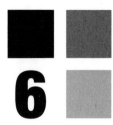

**6**

# Critical Care

The specialty of bariatric critical care is more important than ever as the number of obese and overweight Americans increases. Issues of critical care continue to become increasingly important as larger, heavier people access care on all levels. Excess body weight is a threat to health because it is associated with an increase of cardiovascular disease, type 2 diabetes, hypertension, infertility, stroke, hyperlipidemia, degenerative joint disease, gall stones, and some types of cancers. Excess abdominal adiposity, particularly visceral fat and excess triglyceride content in the liver, skeletal, and heart tissues, is associated with hepatic and skeletal muscle insulin resistance, impaired ventricular function, and increased coronary heart disease.[1] When patients are hospitalized, clinicians must recognize that most very overweight patients are at risk for certain hazards of immobility.[2] Common immobility-related complications include skin breakdown, cardiac deconditioning, deep vein thrombosis, muscle atrophy, urinary stasis, constipation, pain management challenges, and depression. Immobility also contributes to pulmonary complications, such as atelectasis, pneumonia, delayed or traumatic intubation, and exacerbates pre-existing conditions, such as overweight hypoventilation syndrome or sleep apnea. The obese patient is more inclined to develop complications resulting from a long hospitalization.[3]

The implication for critical care clinicians is that managing the patient with these comorbidities is challenging, unpredictable, and requires vigilance in all clinical activities on all levels. When a very overweight person is critically ill, clinicians must recognize that this patient is at risk for certain hazards of immobility. When physically dependent, the obese patient is more inclined to develop complications resulting from a long hospitalization. In critical care, common immobility-related complications could include cardiac deconditioning, deep vein thrombosis, muscle atrophy, urinary stasis, skin breakdown, pain management, depression, and pulmonary concerns. Mobilizing the patient early and safely can reduce some of these immobility-related complications of hospitalization. A variety of strategies are available to promote safe,

### BELLA'S MESSAGE

The rotation therapy provides two important therapeutic modalities in caring for the very overweight patient. The first is prevention of pulmonary complications in the critical care unit; the other is repositioning. Rotation therapy is not usually considered appropriate therapy in prevention or treatment of pressure ulcers among patients who are to be repositioned easily by available staff members. However, many very overweight patients are too difficult to reposition manually. In that situation, rotation therapy may provide a service otherwise not available to the oversized patient.

Consider Bella, a 43-year-old patient admitted to an acute care facility with severe pain of unknown origin. As a result of her severe pain, exacerbated by repositioning, she refused to be turned. Within 10 days of her admission, she developed a stage IV, 10 x 15cm pressure ulcer. At that time, a team conference was called, and it was decided to place the patient on rotation therapy, along with the specially designed mobility equipment. The pressure ulcer took over six months to heal; however, the patient, her family, and clinicians agreed that introduction of the specially designed equipment was a turning point.

The patient was more fully in control of repositioning and, therefore, pain control. She became increasingly more active and, despite her long hospitalization and serious physical illness, was able to transfer from bed to wheelchair. The patient care team effectively matched the patient with the therapeutic modality. Clinicians explain that use of rotation therapy in prevention and treatment of pressure ulcers is often employed in the event that the patient is unable to be turned because of insufficient staff or other reasons, such as if the patient is experiencing severe pain.[9]

size-appropriate patient care, including utilizing appropriate resources, equipment, and criteria-based protocols.

### *RESPIRATORY CONCERNS*

Obesity is associated with altered respiratory function. The incidence of respiratory problems has a direct relationship to body mass index (BMI), meaning the heavier the patient the more likely these problems will occur. Excessive abdominal adiposity mechanically interferes with lung function simply because of the extra weight on the chest wall and rib cage. In addition, obesity is associated with obstructive sleep apnea (OSA) and obesity hypoventilation syndrome (OHS).

OSA is characterized by episodes of apnea and hypopnea during sleep. This is caused by partial or complete upper airway obstruction. Episodes of oxygen desaturation cause transient increase in pulmonary artery and pul-

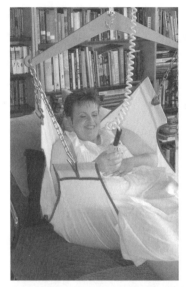

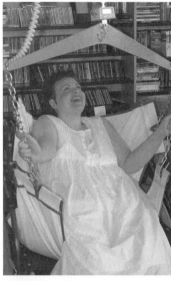

**By providing a patient with specially designed equipment, a patient is more in control of repositioning and can transfer from bed to wheelchair without assistance. This can help prevent pressure ulcers and contribute to overall better quality of life.**

monary wedge pressures, and myocardial perfusion defects. Subsequently, cardiac abnormalities and cardiac rhythm alterations, permanent pulmonary hypertension, right ventricular hypertrophy, and bilateral leg edema can develop.[4]

OHS is common among obese people simply because of their weight. In fact, some authors suggest this condition occurs primarily in the severely obese, or those weighing over 350 pounds. OHS is characterized by episodes of drowsiness, or narcosis, occurring during wake hours, and is caused by abnormalities of breathing and an accumulation of toxic levels of carbon dioxide in the blood. OHS, sometimes referred to as *Pickwickian syndrome*, is a condition related to obstructive sleep apnea, and when it occurs, the very obese person does not breathe a sufficient amount of oxygen during sleep or while awake. The etiology of OHS is thought to involve a combination of factors. First, it is a disorder of the brain's control over breathing, and secondly, the muscles of the chest wall simply are not strong enough to adequately elevate the chest enough to provide adequate expansion to exchange air efficiently. A decreased ability to oxygenate the blood and retention of carbon dioxide occur, leading to chronic respiratory acidosis. This situation leads to progressive symptoms of fatigue, weight gain, poor sleep quality, hypersomnolence, depression, and more. Patients with OHS often exhibit signs of right-sided heart failure.

Right-sided heart failure is seldom a primary condition; rather it is usually a consequence of another medical condition. It is a disorder wherein the right side of the heart loses its ability to pump blood effectively. It is sometimes referred to as congestive heart failure; however this broad term could refer to failure of the right, left or both sides of the heart. Right-sided heart failure occurs in five percent of the population and subsequently leads to congestion affecting the liver, gastrointestinal system, arms and legs, or the lungs. Some of the conditions that lead to right-sided heart failure are obesity with OHS, left-sided heart failure, chronic lung diseases, congenital heart disease, primary pulmonary hypertension, or valve disease. Physical symptoms include swelling of hands and feet, fatigue, weakness, and irregular or rapid heartbeat. Any activity that places additional stress on the body can precipitate symptoms.

Diagnostic tests include electrocardiogram to assess signs of a thickened heart muscle or arrhythmias, echocardiogram to identify enlargement of the heart or other abnormalities, or chest x-ray to determine enlargement of the heart or other cardiopulmonary abnormalities.

Tests performed to confirm a diagnosis of OHS include sleep studies and arterial blood gas analysis. Arterial blood gas analysis, sometimes referred to as blood gases or ABG, measures the acidity, oxygen concentration, and carbon dioxide content of the blood. It is a relatively simple and cost-effective test that is performed to evaluate respiratory diseases and other conditions that affect the lungs or the effectiveness of oxygen therapy. Because of the acid-base component of the test it also provides information on how well the kidneys are functioning. The test is commonly performed by collecting a small sample of arterial blood from the radial, femoral, or brachial artery. Patients report a brief cramping or throbbing at the puncture site. Once the sample is collected, the needle is withdrawn and local pressure is applied for 5 to 10 minutes to prevent unnecessary bleeding or bruising at the site. Patients with OHS are often found to have positive results for respiratory acidosis.

Respiratory acidosis occurs when the lungs fail to remove carbon dioxide. This causes a discrepancy in the acid-base balance, and subsequently body fluids become excessively acidic. In the event of OHS, a mild but chronic impairment of the lung's ability to remove carbon dioxide over a prolonged period of time can lead to very insidious changes. However, when the condition becomes severe it can lead to confusion, irritability, or lethargy. Arterial blood gas analysis can determine the extent of respiratory acidosis.

## AIRWAY PLACEMENT

Airway placement ought to include assessment for the following risk factors: obesity, short or thick neck, facial edema, swollen or thick tongue, receding mandible, protruding/missing maxillary incisors, irregular jaw movement, mandibular size, erratic head and neck movement, and prominence of the upper incisors. Further assessment should include a measurement of the distance from the sternal notch to the tip of the chin in neutral and maximally extended position. With extension, an increase of 5cm should occur. Intubation may prove more challenging, with difficulty visualizing landmarks. The Combitube, an

### THE PROBLEM OF 'TURN Q 2'

If turning and repositioning patients manually accomplishes the same task as specialty beds, it seems logical that the added cost of these automated products is unnecessary. Yet, Krishnagopalan and colleagues set out to determine if this widely accepted standard of care mandating repositioning every two hours was actually met. The research team conducted a survey of nursing personnel regarding patients in a long-term care facility. The study suggested the goals for turning and repositioning dependent patients were not met regardless of practice setting. For example, researchers report, "The result of our study among intensive care specialists was also quite enlightening." Of those subjects responding to the survey, the majority agree the standard is turning every 2 hours, and believe this standard helps prevent the hazards of immobility. However, respondents were less confident the goal was met. Only half of the critical care specialists reported the standard was met 50 percent of the time, even in the presence of a hospital-mandated protocol. So, despite the fact that clinicians understood the mandate and benefit to turning the patient every hour, the task becomes elusive.[11]

esophageal tracheal double lumen airway, is recognized by the American Heart Association and the American Association of Anesthesiologists as an alternative to the endotracheal tube when obesity-related technical difficulties arise.

Failure to control secretions can lead to skin breakdown, malodor, and can threaten a patent airway. The trachea is usually close to the skin surface and easily accessible. For those patients with a thick short neck with excessive parapharyngeal fat deposits, it is often difficult for the surgeon to perform tracheostomy surgery as the trachea may be buried deep in the tissue. A resultant wound must be managed like any other open wound. A nonadhesive, absorbent, quarter-inch foam dressing will absorb excess wound drainage, protect the wound, and prevent injury from adhesives. Tracheostomy ties should be longer and wider to prevent trauma within skin folds.

## MECHANICAL VENTILATION

Due to their high oxygen consumption and poor tolerance for respiratory loads, morbidly obese patients may develop respiratory failure from the most seemingly inconsequential insults. The increased mass of abdominal and thoracic contents alters the lung volumes. A decrease in functional residual capacity (FRC) is seen exponentially with increasing BMI. Expiratory reserve volume and total lung capacity are decreased. FRC may be reduced in the upright position to the extent that it falls within the range of closing capacity with subsequent small airway closure, ventilation perfusion mismatch right to left shunting, and arterial hypoxemia. The reduction of FRC impairs the capacity of obese patients to tolerate apnea. Larger patients desaturate rapidly after induction of anesthesia despite preoxygenation due to smaller oxygen reservoir and increase in oxygen consumption. Residual volume remains normal or slightly increased due to increased air trapping and preexisting obstructive airway disease.

Noninvasive positive-pressure ventilation can be tried before mechanical ventilation is considered. However, mechanical support must be available early and electively. Literature suggests that when treating morbidly obese patients with acute respiratory failure, mechanical ventilation should be initiated with a tidal volume in the range of 5 to 7mL/kg, based on ideal body weight not on actual body weight. Tidal volume should then be titrated to the patient's ventilator mechanics.[5] The concern is that calculating the initial tidal volume on actual body weight can lead to high airway pressure and alveolar distension.

Commonly, the obese patient will experience fatigue of the diaphragmatic muscle. Pressure support ventilation alone or with backup allows for resting of the diaphragm until the state of exhaustion resolves.

## PROPER POSITIONING

Proper positioning can be crucial in critically ill, morbidly obese patients, both to maximize lung function and to increase the likelihood of successful weaning, according to Suzanne M. Burns, RN, MSN, an Associate Professor

### THE THREAT OF SHEARING INJURY

Despite the value of rotation therapy in prevention and treatment of skin injury among the obese patient, it is necessary to take precautions to prevent friction and shear. Correct pressure settings, fitting the patient to the appropriately sized surface, and assessment for skin changes can provide these precautions.[10]

of Nursing at the University of Virginia Health Sciences Center in Charlottesville. Burns reports that in a study of 19 obese patients being weaned from mechanical ventilation, she and her colleagues found that the 45-degree upright and reverse Trendelenburg positions were associated with better respiratory mechanics than were the 90-degree upright and supine positions. Furthermore, patients typically preferred them. "Supine is probably the worst position for these large patients," commented Professor Burns, who explained that the supine position reduces pulmonary compliance and increases airway resistance. "Proning morbidly obese patients is not impossible, just difficult," she added. Evidence suggests that proning can improve functional residual capacity, pulmonary compliance, and oxygenation. Hydraulic lifts, oversized wheelchairs, and other special equipment facilitate positioning of these patients. "A positive attitude and determination on the part of caregivers to position these patients properly despite their size are also essential," she emphasized.[6]

## PNEUMONIA

What is well documented is that pneumonia is the most common cause of death from

> ### ONE NURSE'S ASSESSMENT TOOL
>
> I recognize the importance of diagnostic tools in assessing patients for sleep apnea, but let me share something we do in our office. We have a very active bariatric surgery program, we follow the patients very closely, and we stay acquainted with the most up-to-date methods for screening patients for respiratory pathology. Yet, recently we tried something we found to be simple, inexpensive, and maybe even innovative. The receptionist in the lobby reported that she was surprised at how many of our patients drifted off to sleep while in the waiting room. She noted that many of the patients who fell asleep often began breathing very loudly while they slept. Based on this observation, she was asked to report which patients fell asleep and which patients also "snored" loudly. Since we know that obese patients have a higher than average incidence of sleep apnea, we know statistically our patients are at a greater risk. We also know that patients with sleep apnea are seldom rested and frequently doze off during waking hours. We suspected this might happen even when waiting 10 to 15 minutes for an appointment. Certainly, this is not scientifically based or diagnostic, but it does raise a red flag as to which of our patients may have sleep apnea, which in turn helps us to treat our patients more effectively with better outcome.

nosocomial infection. The prevalence of hospital-acquired pneumonia is 5 to 10 per 1,000 admissions. Although nosocomial pneumonia can develop in any hospitalized patient, it occurs fourfold in patients receiving mechanical ventilation. In the recumbent position, tidal volume diminishes during sleep and mucociliary transport is decreased; both can result in atelectasis to varying degrees and can lead to lower respiratory tract complications. Infectious and inflammatory complications of the lower respiratory tract lead to increased mortality, morbidity, and cost in the intubated,

ventilated patient who is critically ill.

Early and comprehensive assessment, prevention, and intervention are essential in managing this complex clinical situation. The patient with pneumonia should be assessed for the etiology and severity of the pneumonia. The patient most at risk for pneumonia is the immobile, institutionalized patient with multisystem involvement and a history of recurrent pneumonia. Patients with nasogastric tube feedings are at significant risk for aspiration pneumonia, especially in the presence of elevated intra-abdominal pressure, such as

## THE PROBLEM OF SLEEP

**The problem is that people who are obese and nap tend to fall asleep faster and sleep longer during the day. Research suggests that at night, however, it takes longer to fall asleep and they sleep less than people of normal weight. In an apparent vicious cycle, recent studies indicate that not only can obesity interfere with sleep, but that sleep problems may actually contribute to obesity. This type of sleep disturbance is largely due to obstructive sleep apnea, which is characterized by episodes of drowsiness, or narcosis, occurring during wake hours, and is caused by abnormalities of breathing and an accumulation of toxic levels of carbon dioxide in the blood.**

seen among morbidly obese patients. In making a diagnosis, a chest x-ray demonstrates aspirate in the lungs and the onset and location of infiltrate. The clinical manifestation of pneumonia is elevated temperature, chest congestion, and decreased lung sounds, and the patient will appear acutely ill.

## *ROTATION THERAPY*

With increasing interest in rotation therapy for purposes of preventing pneumonia, skin injury, and caregiver injury, it becomes more important to fully understand the meaning of terminology pertaining to this therapy, its cost, and indication. Questions need to be asked to determine the actual value of this emerging and evolving therapy. The principal behind this form of kinetic therapy is patient movement. Therapies fall into one of two categories: one rotates, in log-roll fashion, the entire body. This is commonly referred to as full-body lateral rotation (FBLRT). The other main category of rotation therapy moves the torso. This is commonly referred to as continuous lateral rotation therapy (CLRT). FBLRT is thought to take rotation therapy a step beyond CLRT in that as the name indicates the entire body is turned in a log roll-type manner. Like CLRT, this does not substitute for repositioning the patient, but unlike CLRT, FBLRT provides a full turn of the entire body and is thought to address not only pulmonary issues, but also skin injury. Some clinicians use FBLRT for their patients where frequent turning becomes a problem whether because of staffing concerns, fear of caregiver injury, or the size and weight distribution of the patient.

A number of researchers are looking at strategies for improving clinical and cost outcomes with the use of rotation therapy in the critical care areas. One such study recognized that the use of rotation therapy for patients with risk of pneumonia and other respiratory problems had increased in their respective organization in the previous 10 years, largely because of more research and improved products. Cost and clinical challenges emerged with this increased utilization. The researchers introduced two separate but related interdisciplinary teams to address the cost and clinical aspects of rotation therapy. Changes were introduced and outcomes improved dramatically. For example, more patients used the therapy; however, the total bed days were decreased, as was a decrease in CRLT length of stay (LOS) and ICU LOS. This study suggested that timely and appropriate use of rotation therapy was one method to control costs and improve patient care.[7]

With continued interest in the benefits and burdens of advanced technology, clinicians increasingly seek methods to determine the clinical and cost value of such technology. Kathleen Wright recently described the importance of developing criteria for using certain advanced

## OBESITY AND DEEP VEIN THROMBOSIS

**A** BMI >29 heightens the prevalence of pulmonary embolism. Deep vein thrombosis (DVT) appears twice as often in obese patients as it does in their nonobese counterparts. Thromboembolic events are the most common complications of bariatric surgery, with an incidence of 2.4 to 4.5 percent due to prolonged immobility, venous stasis, polycythemia (which is associated with OHS) and intra-abdominal pressure, which increases pressure on the deep veins.

technologies, such as rotation therapy. She reports a study involving 44 patients, all meeting placement criteria for therapy. Study patients averaged 10 days of therapy versus the national average of 16 days. Twenty-one patients received therapy for prevention of pneumonia/adult respiratory distress syndrome (ARDS), 16 with a positive outcome. Twenty-seven patients were placed on therapy for pneumonia/ARDS, and 17 achieved a positive outcome. At a daily rental cost of $135, with 210 total prevention-therapy days, the total cost of prevention/treatment was $28,350. With a mean incremental cost of pneumonia treatment at $13,400, and 16 pneumonia cases avoided, total savings equaled $93,800. Subtract the rental costs from the cost-avoidance and the total savings was $65,450. How was this accomplished? The researcher presents a criteria-based protocol to begin

therapy, criteria for discontinuing therapy, education, competencies, and continued monitoring of equipment.[8]

## THE SKIN

Most clinical experts agree that a relationship exists between skin injury, wound healing, and immobility. The stress of the pneumonia threatens the wound healing, as do other hazards of immobility, such as pain, cardiac deconditioning, and embolic processes. Wounds are particularly sensitive to pneumonia and will generally plateau, fail to progress, or deteriorate until the pneumonia resolves. Prevention of wound trauma and further skin breakdown are expected outcomes for the immobile patient with pneumonia and skin injury. Timely, appropriate introduction of FBLRT may best serve the patient in reducing interface pressures, promoting pulmonary function, and providing therapeutic positioning.[3]

## EQUIPMENT

Airway management requires special thought to equipment, intubation, securing the airway, secretion control, and proper positioning. Take care to tailor equipment to best serve the actual needs of the patient and caregivers. Products that could promote critical care include Combitube, Portex USA tracheostomy tube, a wider, longer tracheostomy tube holder, wheelchairs, walkers, frame with support surface, trapeze, longer gloves, lateral transfer device, abdominal binder, arm board, nasogastric tube holder, gown, sequential compression device, peripherally inserted central catheter, and intravenous arm board.

## SUMMARY

As with many normal-weight patients, an increased length of stay can lead to immobility and deconditioning in the obese patient. In addition, the obese patient may have pre-existing emotional concerns, which manifest as fear or reluctance to participate. Passive behaviors, or perhaps anger and acting out, are sometimes observed. Caregivers express reluctance to provide manual lifting and moving because of the realistic fear of personal injury. All these factors and the presence of critical illness place the patient at risk for common, predictable, and costly complications. An interdisciplinary team comprises psychologists, social workers, ergonomists, physical/occupational therapists, and others and may address some of the concerns associated with an increased length of stay.

## REFERENCES

1.  Alpert MA. Obesity cardiomyopathy: Pathophysiology and evolution of the clinical syndrome. *Am J Med Sci* 2001;321:225–36.
2.  Gallagher S, Arouzman J, Lacovara J, et al. Criteria-based protocols and the obese patient: Planning care for a high risk population. *Ostomy Wound Manage* 2004;50(6):32–8.
4.  Marrone O, Bonsignore MR. Pulmonary hemodynamics in obstructive sleep apnea. *Sleep Med Rev* 2002;6;175–93.
5.  Begany T. ICU management of the morbidly obese. *Pulmonary Reviews.Com* 2002;7(4):1–5.
6.  Burns SM, Egloff MB, Ryan B, et al. Effect of body position on spontaneous respiratory rate and tidal volume in patients with obesity, abdominal distension and ascites. *Am J Crit Care* 1994;3:102–6.
7.  Weinberg KA, Kaplon SB, Johansen S, Ruhren CA. Process improvement: Use of continuous lateral rotation therapy. *Crit Care Med* 1999;27(1):51suppl.
8.  Wright KD. Justifying CLRT implementation. *Nurs Manage* 2003;34(8):56A–56D.
3.  Sussman C, Bates-Jensen B. *Wound Care: A Collaborative Practice Manual for Physical Therapists and Nurses.* Gaithersburg, MD: Aspen Publishers, 1998.
9.  Gallagher S. Continuous lateral rotation therapy in the bariatric patient. *XTRAWise* 2000;2(1).
10. Panniculectomy: Not just a tummy tuck. *Nursing* 2004;03(12).
11. Krishnagopalan S, Johnson EW, Low LL, Kaufman L. Body positioning of intensive care patients: Clinical practice versus standards. *Crit Care Med* 2002;30(11):2588–92.

# Skin Injury

The skin is the largest organ of the body, both by weight and by surface area, accounting for 16 percent of the total body weight. Unfortunately, despite efforts at preventing skin injury, occasionally skin is injured, and when injury occurs, it triggers a cascade of untoward events. Aggressive intervention is necessary to manage skin injury among obese patients. However, this can be complex in many respects. The skin, wounds, assessment, intervention, and outcomes are described, all within a holistic framework.

## THE SKIN

The skin is comprised of two main layers: the epidermis and the dermis. The dermis is tough, flexible, and elastic in most people. The highly vascular dermis contains the lymphatics, epithelial cells, connective tissue, muscle, fat, and nerve tissue. Hair follicles and sebaceous and sweat glands, which are located in the dermis, contribute epithelial cells for rapid reepithelization of partial-thickness wounds. The sebaceous glands are responsible for secretions that lubri-

## PULSED LAVAGE

Pulsatile jet irrigators or pulsed lavage therapy are commonly, but cautiously, used for debridement.[16] The system is best described as a suction lavage device that uses pressure-pulsed irrigation and suction to remove debris and bacteria from wounds. All of the systems available today provide a pistol-style handpiece with triggers to control to pulsatile force. The advantage of this therapy is that it can be delivered by nursing staff, physical therapy staff, and others at the bedside.[17] The disadvantage is the risk of infections related to the treatment. According to one study, pulsed lavage therapy can scatter infections up to 8 feet. A recent article published in *Nursing 2005* addresses these issues, explaining that standard precautions must be followed, personal protective equipment must be in place, and the treatment room must be cleaned between patients. More specifically, consider the following precautions.

1. Use continuous suction, keeping the splash guard in place at all times.
2. Empty the canister after each use.
3. Perform the procedure in a private, enclosed, properly ventilated room.
4. Cover any surfaces that could be contaminated with aerosol.
5. Wear water proof gown, gloves, mask, face shield, and eye and hair cover.
6. Cover any patient wound not being treated.
7. After treatment thoroughly clean and disinfect all surfaces.[18]

cate the skin and keep it soft and pliable. The sweat gland secretions control skin pH to prevent dermal infections. The sweat glands, dermal blood vessels, and small muscles in the skin control the body's surface temperature. The nerve endings in the skin include receptors for pain, touch, heat, and cold. Loss of the nerve endings in the skin increases risk for skin injury by failing to provide these protective mechanisms and by decreasing the tolerance of the tis-

sues to external forces.

The deep layer of the dermis merges with the subcutaneous fat and fascia and may be confused with yellow slough, so this may require careful evaluation for texture and vitality, especially when selecting treatment modalities discussed later. The dermis is more resistant to pressure than underlying soft tissue, so pressure injury can occur deep within the tissues before breakdown as the skin level becomes evident.

The vascular supply of the dermis nourishes the epidermis, which is the outer most layer of the skin. This avascular structure is about as thick as a piece of paper. New skin cells grow at the base of the epidermis. These cells push their way to the surface where they will eventually slough away.

The skin then functions as a barrier, as a communication modality, as a sensory, thermoregulatory, and immunologic organ. Loss of skin integrity can mean infection, pain, malodor, loss of independence, and loss of self esteem.

## UNDERSTANDING OUTCOMES

Although healthcare clinicians have always paid attention to the way their care influences the patient, now clinicians are being rewarded for achieving clinical results. While changes in reimbursement practices have influenced this practice to some extent, the practice of rewarding clinicians for achievement of clinical results is mainly due to the recent outcomes movement. For instance, instead of simply providing service, the successful clinician seeks wound resolution before capitated funds are used up; therefore, meaningful clinical, cost, and satisfaction outcomes are achieved.

Once the clinical diagnosis

is established, the clinician is asked to predict the expected outcome goals and select the most appropriate intervention. Prediction and prognosis are useful tools for outcome management. However, many clinicians are intimidated by the idea of predicting outcomes. This might be because clinicians must be very familiar and comfortable with the effects of the interventions they select in order to make this prediction. Further, the obese patient may achieve unpredictable results. Yet today caregivers are able to more accurately predicts outcomes for the patient, payers, and themselves. In the current healthcare environment, familiarity with outcomes is important for all stakeholders involved with care. Therefore, assessment drives outcomes and outcomes drive intervention. A thorough understanding of assessment, including common types of skin injury, is critical to outcome management.

## PREVENTING PRESSURE ULCERS

Pressure ulcers are a direct result of pressure, friction, and shear. Factors contributing to pressure ulcers include moisture, dehydration, malnutrition, and immobility. Pressure

ulcers typically occur over bony prominences and develop because of the inability to adequately reposition the patient from that area. The inability to adequately reposition patients is a significant concern especially among obese patients. In addition, larger, heavier patients can be at risk for atypical or unusual pressure ulcers, which occur due to pressure within skin folds, as a result of tubes or catheters, or from an ill-fitting chair or wheelchair.

For instance, pressure within skin folds can be sufficient to cause skin breakdown. Tubes and catheters burrow into skin folds, especially if the tissue is edematous or cellulitic. This causes erosion of the skin surface. Pressure from side rails and armrests not designed to accommodate a larger person can cause pressure ulcers on the patient's hips and trunk/torso. Atypical skin breakdown can be minimized by using properly sized equipment. Additionally, the patient needs to be repositioned at least every two hours, as do tubes and catheters. Tubes should be placed so that the patient does not rest on them. Tube/catheter holders may be helpful in this step.

Many obese patients have large panniculuses, some

weighing as much as 50 pounds. The abdominal panniculus must be repositioned in order to prevent pressure injury. Alert patients are usually able to lift the pannus off of the suprapubic area or describe to clinicians the manner in which the patient prevented injury at home. If clinically appropriate, the dependent, weak or unconscious patient can be placed in the side-lying position and the nurse can lift the pannus away from the underlying skin surface allowing air to flow to the regions, while relieving pressure. Rotation therapy is available to ensure sufficient repositioning for a very large patient who otherwise may pose a realistic challenge to frequent turning. Despite the value of rotation therapy in prevention and treatment of skin injury in the obese patient, it is necessary to take precautions to prevent friction and shear, e.g., correct pressure settings, appropriately sized surface areas on beds, tables, and chairs, and assessment for skin changes.[1]

## CANDIDIASIS

Diabetes mellitus places the patient at risk for candidiasis. The combination of obesity and diabetes places the patient at great risk, especially in the presence of excess moisture from urine, perspiration, or wound drainage. *Candida albicans* is the most common source of human infection; it is a yeast-like fungus that thrives in a dark, moist environment, affecting primarily the intertriginous areas.[2] In addition to diabetes mellitus, other factors that contribute to candidiasis include immunosuppression, systemic infection, chronic steroid and antibiotic use, hyperhidrosis, and obesity. Many obese patients report chronic candidal involvement within skin folds. When an obese patient is hospitalized, moisture from urine, perspiration, or wound drainage exacerbates this chronic but otherwise mild condition. Clinically, candidiasis is characterized by scaling erythema, and in some cases small pustules or pus-filled lesions may appear. Patients often complain of itching or burning. If the condition progresses without intervention, it could lead to death. More commonly, however, candidiasis leads to fissuring and maceration. Further, in the face of associated pruritus, patients may scratch the skin surface, further compromising skin integrity, which can lead to a secondary bacterial invasion.

Prevention includes blood sugar control, use of cotton undergarments, avoiding tight clothing, and avoiding unnecessary antibiotic or steroid use. In the event prevention fails, the first objective is to eliminate excessive moisture to the skin surface. Locally, if the patient reports a moist skin surface, initially, an antifungal powder can be applied to clean, completely dry skin. For a dry, flaking surface, an antifungal cream can be helpful. To help soothe and cleanse affected skin, a soak or compress of Burow's solution (aluminum acetate) can be applied for 15 to 20 minutes twice a day. Others suggest use of a one-percent acetic acid (10mL of vinegar to 1 quart of water) solution as a soak or compress.[3] If the condition does not improve within 24 hours, consider reassessing the condition because many skin conditions mimic others.

## INCONTINENCE DERMATITIS

Moisture and chemical irritants often lead to skin injury; therefore, incontinence often leads to dermatitis. Predisposing factors for urinary incontinence and subsequently dermatitis include gender, genetics, race, culture, neurology, anatomy, and collagen status. Urinary incontinence is greater in women, regardless of age. Studies independent of age suggest a direct correlation between increased body mass index (BMI) and urinary incontinence.[4] Sleep apnea, a condition associated with obesity, leads to decreased oxygen tension and relative central nervous system hypoxia. Both of these clinical conditions cause increased excitability of autonomic neurons. Urgency, urge incontinence, and enuresis can be improved with continuous positive pressure.[5]

In the acute care setting, many otherwise continent patients develop short-term incontinence when physically dependent. This may occur because of medication, a delay in locating enough caregivers to place the patient on the bedpan, or simply because the patient can't reach a commode in time to prevent an incontinent episode. Also, patients are frequently reluctant to ask for assistance with hygiene. Patients need to be reminded that our goal is to serve their needs. Maintaining clean, dry skin is our objective, and if the patient needs assistance in this effort, caregivers are available to help.

After each incontinent episode, clean the entire affected area with a deodorizing incontinence cleanser, and then rinse if indicated. Patients report that drying the buttocks, perineal area, and between folds with an institutionally approved blow dryer on the cool setting is more comfortable than towel drying. If the patient is able, he or she may prefer to perform this personal care him- or her-self. Regardless, this technique for drying the area may be less traumatic to the outer most layer of skin and may reduce the threat of cutaneous cross contamination.

In the presence of inconti-nence dermatitis, a therapeu-tic moisture barrier ointment can serve as a protective bar-rier to chemicals in urine or stool. Few moisture barrier ointments adhere to weeping or moist areas of superficial breakdown. A light coat of protective powder applied to the moist areas may increase adherence of the moisture barrier ointment, thus more completely protecting the skin surface from the irritat-ing chemicals found in stool and urine. Failure to provide clinicians with properly fit-ting gloves could serve as a barrier to adequate cleansing. Most organizations have access to elbow length gloves, which provide for employee protection and patient dignity.

## LEGS AND FEET

Many obese people report foot pain. This might be because the feet carry the

---

**OUTFITTING AN OUTPATIENT WOUND CENTER**

Consider the waiting area: Use sturdy armless chairs and high, firm sofas. In the exam area, a sturdy exam table should be available that is bolted to the floor to prevent tipping, and larger gowns, blood pressure cuffs, and drapes should be available for the patients. Keep all specialized equipment in one easy-to-locate area. Never place scales in a public area.[19] If the center is serving large numbers of obese patients, consider publications specifically written for larger people. And don't forget! Always ask your patients what you can do to help them feel more comfortable.

---

patient's entire weight; there-fore, heavier people are prone to wear and tear injuries as some activities can exert up to four times the body's weight. Foot care, especially among the obese population, requires special attention. Foot pain can sig-nal serious medical condi-tions, such as arthritis, nerve and circulatory disorders, or diabetes. Patients should be reminded that a podiatry con-sultation is important in the presence of foot or ankle pain. Medication, physical therapy, exercise, orthotics, braces, specially designed shoes, and surgery are among the tools used to relieve pain and restore feet to as near normal function as possible.[6]

In the event of skin injury, patients receiving outpatient services for wound care may find something as simple as transportation challenging, and once the patient arrives in the outpatient setting, the physical environment may pose a barrier to care.

Consider accommodation in the physical environment that promotes patient safety, dignity, and comfort.

## THE SURGICAL EXPERIENCE

Hospitalization, including the surgical experience, pre-disposes the patient to skin injury simply because surgery increases the patient's length of stay and dependency or immobility because of pain, sedation, or the fear of falling.[7] Transfers from the operating room table require extra personnel and support-ive equipment, taking care not to create shearing injury or place undue stress on inci-sions.[8] A lateral transfer device may help.

Some patients will fail to progress postoperatively either because of surgical complications or a critical condition. Unless the patient can be mobilized in critical care, deconditioning can occur very rapidly and, there-fore, create a greater risk for skin and wound-related complications.[9] A physical therapy consultation within 24 hours of an ICU admission may be valuable to 1) evaluate for and demonstrate immobility-related equipment, and 2) offer passive activities and exercises with the aim of reducing problems associated with deconditioning.

Postoperatively, patients seem to breathe more easily when the bed is at 30 degrees, because this position prevents the weight of the abdominal adipose tissue from pressing against the diaphragm.[10] The challenge this poses in terms of skin care is that patients who fear shortness of breath may refuse repositioning from this 30-degree semi-Fowler's position, thus placing them at risk for sacral pressure injury. Introducing a therapeutic support surface early in the admission may reduce some of this risk.

Surgical wounds healing by primary intention are expected to create a watertight seal within 24 hours; however, wound healing can be delayed in some obese patients because of interference with the normal wound healing process. Wounds dehisce due to direct tension to the wound. In addition, blood supply to fatty tissue may be insufficient to provide an adequate amount of oxy-

## CARING FOR THE LEGS AND FEET

### Toenails
- Trim toenails as they natural grow, not necessarily straight across.
- If an infection secondary to an ingrown toenail develops, a professional should remove that side of the nail to resolve the infection.
- Fungal nails are common and should be soaked in a 1:1 vinegar/water solution for 20 minutes, with antifungal solution applied afterwards. Oral antifungal medications, specifically Conazoles, may be toxic to the liver and do not always provide long-term relief.
- Consider routine foot care every three months with a podiatrist or skilled practitioner. Meticulous nail care decreases the vector for inflammation and infection.

### Toes
- The inner spaces between the toes need to be kept clean and dry.
- Soaking in a 1:1 vinegar/water solution as tolerated for 20 minutes at least once a week and running a piece of gauze between the toes to remove any debris/detritus will help promote healthy web spaces.
- Using a drying agent/antifungal solution will decrease chances of maceration, irritation, and infection.
- Applying natural lamb's wool between the toes allows the web greater breathability.
- Open toed compression garments will also allow greater breathability, as will breathable footwear that is fitted correctly.

### Proper footwear
- Fitting proper footwear can be a problem. Shoes should be selected at the time of the day when the feet are most swollen, which is at the end of the day for most people.
- If compression garments are worn, make sure the shoes accommodate for this.
- A lace-up or Velcro-strap shoe allows greater accommodation.
- Good athletic shoes are usually larger in the toe box, more supportive, and more breathable. New Balance and Sketchers are two examples of brands with wider sizes.
- Never compromise the length fit to accommodate the width.
- Men's shoes are generally wider. You can find dress shoes that have extra depth and width using a shoe repair shop, prosthetist, orthotist, or podiatrist. These shoes can be sized and ordered without having to be custom made. For very large feet, a Velcro-strap shoe is usually more accommodating.
- Bunions, hammertoes, corns, and calluses are a consequence of biomechanical/functional faults in your inherited foot type. Improper footgear exacerbates the symptoms.

**CARING FOR THE LEGS AND FEET (Continued)**

*Orthotics and proper alignment*
- Using an orthotic, which is an insert that cups the heel and balances the forefoot, can help redistribute weight more correctly.
- Utilizing a heel lift, a piece of felt cut to support heel regions, can help increase range of motion at the ankles and help correct a functional leg length discrepancy, both synergistically supporting better foot function.
- Heel lifts and good functional orthotics coupled with correctly fitted footgear are essential to good mechanics and are the foundation for better postural alignment.
- If the patient already has foot pathology, such as a bunion or hammertoes, further inserts and shoe modification are also important.
- The irritation from improper shoe fit can cause stress, cellulitis/lymphangitis, vectors for infection, corns, and calluses.

*Foot pathology and surgery*
Corns and calluses should be trimmed by a podiatrist or skilled practitioner on a routine basis. Never use any callous removal pads, as they have the potential to cause burns and infections. Foot pathology can only be treated once the cause is understood—this is the value of having professionals involved in care.

gen and nutrients.[11] This too interferes with wound healing. Wound healing may also be delayed if the patient has a diet that lacks essential vitamins and nutrients or if the wound is within a skin fold where excess moisture and bacteria can accumulate. Further, excess abdominal fat increases tension at the wound edges.[12] To reduce the occurrence of abdominal wound separation, some clinicians use a surgical binder to support the area; however, safety considerations need to be addressed when using a binder. The binder should rest no higher than 4cm below the xiphoid process, with at least 2.5cm between the skin and the binder. The binder will need to be large enough to safely meet these needs. Binders are especially important when the patient ambulates. Some patients find the binders so comfortable that they ask to leave the binder on at all times. Careful assessment under the binder will reveal any signs of early pressure-related breakdown where the edges of the binder meet the skin.

Respiratory challenges are common among obese patients.[13] If long-term ventilator support becomes necessary, performing a tracheostomy can be especially challenging if the trachea is buried deep within fatty tissue. A large wound may be needed in order to locate the trachea. This larger wound can lead to complications, such as bleeding, infection, or damage to the surrounding tissue. Postoperative tracheostomy care, therefore, must include steps to protect the peristomal skin, manage the tracheostomy, and contain wound drainage. Locally, a nonadhesive, moisture-absorbing dressing is helpful in achieving this goal.[14] To compound this dilemma, standard-sized trachea tubes may be inadequate for use in patients with larger necks. In addition, narrow cloth trach ties can burrow deep within the folds of neck, causing further damage to the skin. The thicker or wider ties have been used by clinicians to prevent this sort of damage.

## WOUNDS AND WOUND HEALING

Wounds can be acute or chronic with a variety of etiologies, including diabetes-related breakdown, pressure ulcers, arterial or venous wounds, lymphatic wounds, or surgical sites. Wounds can be full or partial thickness. Partial-thickness wounds are superficial and manifest clinically as a blister or abrasion. Full-thickness wounds can extend into muscle, bone, vasculature, or tendon.

As normal acute wounds heal, there is an orderly progression through the wound healing phases, which are inflammation, proliferation, epithelialization, and remodeling.

Failure of an orderly progression through these phases of wound healing will result in a chronic wound. The chronic wound may fail to initiate or may stop progressing in any of the four phases of wound healing. When a wound plateaus in any one of the wound phases, the wound is likely to become chronic (i.e., stuck in that particular phase of healing). For example, a blister within an abdominal skin fold could plateau in the inflammatory phase of wound healing, thus the term *chronic inflammation*. On the other hand, consider the wound that continues to fill with granulation tissue. The proliferation phase proceeds unchecked and the body goes on to form hypergranulation tissue. This is termed chronic proliferation. Or consider the common example of the wound with impaired scarring, such as with hypertrophic scars or keloid formation. A wound in this condition does not stop laying down collagen. This is

termed chronic epithelialization. Topical products may help control hypertrophic scars.

The wound that fails to pass through one of the wound healing phases is lacking attributes of that phase, and this is referred to as absence of inflammation, absence of proliferation, or absence of epithelialization. For instance, those wounds that fail to mount an inflammatory response will not demonstrate signs of inflammation, whereas wounds with chronic inflammation will show signs of a continued inflammatory response. Absence of the wound healing phase signifies either the inability to heal normally or the need for help from an external intervention to initiate the acute phase leading to progression through phases, such as aggressive debridement, introduction of a growth factor ,or surgical revascularization.

## A HOLISTIC APPROACH TO ASSESSMENT

Assessment is the first step in understanding chronic wounds among obese patients. A holistic understanding of the patient is best accomplished by assessing the patient's sociologic, economic, psychologic, and cultural histories; therefore, a complete history and physical

examination are important data gathering tools in this step. The time spent conducting the history and physical provides the clinician a valuable opportunity to begin to develop the therapeutic relationship with a particular patient. Assessment-based intervention of the patient's wound problem is best accomplished within a holistic context.

It is easier to plan appropriate care with a complete history. Patient history is commonly achieved through an interview process, which could include input from the patient, family member(s), caregivers, significant others, or the past medical record. Past and current comorbidities are important to define.

Questions need to be asked, such as, "What co-existing diagnoses or obesity-related comorbidities might impact wound healing?" An understanding of family health history may serve as an important indicator of risk factors. Sleep and activity patterns could influence healing. Many obese people have obesity-related respiratory problems and either fail to use equipment designed to improve ventilation or simply do not have access to these resources. Regardless, it becomes important to identify this as part of a complete history. Identifying prescription and over-the-counter medications can be helpful because some medications interfere with wound healing. Obese patients may regularly use over-the counter drugs such as laxatives, diuretics, or weight loss drinks or pills. Ask about dosages, frequency, adherence with medication regime, the patient's understanding for taking the medication, and how the medication influences wound healing. Regular activity is thought to promote circulation and improve blood sugar; on the other hand, long periods of standing could lead to exacerbations of certain types of wounds. Smoking tobacco or other substances can alter microcirculation and thus should be identified early on. The goal of the history is to better understand the patient's activities and habits and how these affect outcomes. Patients must feel comfortable with the clinicians to confide very personal information.

Nutrition plays a significant role in wound healing. Determine recent changes in patient's weight because weight loss is thought to predict poor wound healing. Recent weight loss may be due to an unbalanced or fad/extreme diet. Many overweight people are familiar with every fad diet, but fail to understand balanced nutri-

tion and its role in health and wound healing. Identify the patient's usual daily food intake. Ask the patient to keep a log to better evaluate a sample of what he or she might eat in a 24-hour period. The clinician can review with the patient the intake of fruits, vegetables, meats, dairy products, and breads and cereals, looking for high-risk food behaviors, such as high intake of fatty foods, low intake of fiber, fruits, and vegetables, or high intake of food with little to no nutritional value.

Sometimes a chronic wound affects the entire family structure, impacting the role of the patient within the family structure. Wounds can be costly, affecting economic and time resources available to the family unit. Any chronic illness or condition can have a psychologic effect on the patient and each of the family members. Wounds hold different meanings to different people and different cultural groups. It is important for the clinician to understand the meaning of being an obese person with a chronic wound.

A thorough physical assessment may be difficult to perform as exam tables may be inadequate for larger patients. Yet it is important as it provides further information on comorbidities that

may impair wound healing. The individual's capacity to heal may be limited by the effects certain diseases have on tissue integrity, perfusion, mobility, adherence, nutrition, and risk for wound infection. Throughout the patient history and physical assessment, the savvy clinician looks for those factors that could influence the wound healing process. These factors will influence the need for more invasive assessment, diagnosis, therapeutic intervention, clinical experts, and ultimately outcomes. For example, obstructive sleep apnea, a common condition among obese people, can interfere with oxygenation. Consider the patient with severe osteoarthritis with limited mobility and resources. Regardless of the physical, social, emotional, or cultural comorbidities, it best serves the patient when the clinician addresses the factors that contribute to wound formation and result in wound healing delays.

Skin changes are important predictors of the body's ability to respond to injury; therefore, the wound and periwound area give clues to more fully understanding the wound. These areas reveal the health of the skin, the phase of wound healing, and the patient's overall health status. In assessing the skin around the wound, assess for predictors of delayed wound healing, such as a distorted anatomy of the skin; skin texture, which can be dry, thick, or of poor turgor; the presence of scar tissue, folds maceration, edema, and discoloration; alterations in sensation, which includes pain, thermal, tough, or protective sensation; skin temperature, hair maldistribution; problems with the toenails; or the presence of blisters. The presence of any these conditions could delay healing and therefore influence wound healing outcomes. In addition to periwound assessment, important wound characteristics are location, depth, color(s) of the wound bed, presence of moisture, malodor, tenderness, and staging or classification.

At the present time, a variety of wound classification systems are used to describe wound severity. Although the classification systems were designed and researched with one specific wound type, they are often inappropriately used for any wound type. Wound classification systems could include classifying surgical wounds, severity scoring of lower leg ulcers, diabetes-related ulcerations, and so on. For example, the National Pressure Ulcer Advisory Panel (NPUAP) pressure

ulcer staging criteria was developed for use with pressure ulcers, the Wagner staging system was developed for grading the severity of dysvascular ulcers, and the Marion Laboratories color system was developed to grade ulcer severity based on color (red/black/yellow).Each of these systems are appropriate in classifying certain types of wounds.

The NPUAP pressure ulcer staging system and the Wagner staging system are classifications based on tissue layers and depth of tissue destruction. The partial-thickness and full-thickness skin loss classifications are tissue layer descriptions of skin loss. Marion Laboratories, in Europe, developed a system based on the color of the wound surface, which simply put will be red, yellow, or black. Red is thought to suggest the wound is healthy, requiring protection to move on through the healing phases. Yellow denotes the wound is covered with a type of necrotic slough and requires aggressive cleaning. Black refers to a necrotic wound that requires debridement of the necrotic matter.

In addition to the classification/staging systems, it is valuable to include wound characteristics because no wound classification system

when used in isolation is an appropriate method of measuring wound healing or outcome potential. The NPUAP Pressure Ulcer Staging System uses a classification by stages to describe the anatomic depth of soft tissue damage and is designed for use in wounds with a pressure or tissue perfusion etiology. The pressure ulcer staging system must be used in conjunction with other wound assessment parameters because it does not describe the wound. This staging system is widely accepted and commonly used to communicate wound severity, to organize treatment protocols, and to select and be reimbursed for treatment products for pressure ulcers.

The presence of wound drainage is another important wound assessment parameter because the characteristics of the exudate helps the clinician diagnose wound infection, evaluate effectiveness of local treatment, and monitor wound healing outcomes. Attention must be given to wound infection because a high bacterial load delays wound healing. Proper assessment of wound exudates is also important because it affirms the body's brief, normal, inflammatory response to tissue injury. Thus, accurate assessment of wound exudates and diagnosis of infection are critical components of effective wound management.

The healthy wound normally has some evidence of moisture. Healthy wound fluid contains enzymes and growth factors, which may play a role in promoting reepithelization of the wound and provide needed growth factors for all phases of wound repair. The moist environment allows efficient migration of epidermal cells and prevents wound desiccation and further injury.

In acute wounds healing by primary intention, exudate on the incision is normal during the first 48 to 72 hours. After that time, the presence of exudate is a sign of impaired healing. Infection and seroma are the two most likely causes. In chronic wounds, increased exudates are a response to the inflammatory process or infection. The capillary becomes increasingly permeable and fluid escapes into the wound. Evaluation of the wound type, the number and type of organisms present, and the condition of the patient are important in determining risk for infection. Evaluation of wound type includes assessment of acute versus chronic wounds and necrotic versus clean, nonhealing wounds. The number and type of

organisms present in the wound are evaluated for burden on the wound, possible bacteria-produced toxins, and pathology of the organisms. A holistic approach emphasizes an assessment of the patient's overall condition as it relates to immune function.

If the wound becomes infected, the wound drainage changes. For example, a thick, malodorous, sweet-smelling, green drainage suggests the presence of pseudomonas organisms. In the event of a proteus infection, an ammonia odor may develop. Wounds with foul-smelling drainage are generally infected or filled necrotic debris and will often have thick, tenacious, purulent, malodorous drainage in moderate to copious amounts. Wound exudate should be differentiated from necrotic tissue, which is easily eliminated with effective debridement. Exudate from sloughing necrotic tissue is commonly attached to or connected with the necrotic debris. However, frequently the only method of differentiation is adequate debridement of necrotic tissue from the wound.

Local signs of wound infection include erythema or skin discoloration, edema, warmth, induration, increased pain, and purulent drainage with or without a

foul odor. Systemic signs of infection include elevated temperature, elevated white blood cell count, and confusion in the older adult.

Clean wounds are contaminated with bacteria but usually progress through wound healing uneventfully. If the wound fails to progress, even in the presence of appropriate intervention, the patient may have an occult infection. An occult infection is suspected when colony counts rise above 100,000 organisms per millimeter while there are little to no empirical indicators of infection. Control of a high bioburden is essential before other interventions should be considered.

## THERAPEUTIC INTERVENTION

A holistic approach to obesity-related wound care manages comorbidities that influence wound healing. For instance, attention to protein nutrition, inactivity, readjustment of medications, or control of bioburden within skin folds might improve wound healing potential.

Many times patients and clinicians over-treat acute and chronic wounds. It is of great concern as excessive intervention can be as harmful as the failure to intervene. For example, aggressive cleansing with cytotoxic agents can delay healing as seriously as a failure to recognize occult bacterial invasion. Protect clean, superficial wounds. Recognize the maxim, "Do No Harm," in everyday practice, aligning treatment with wound characteristics.

Wound cleansers can be critical to reducing bacterial load, and must be used prior to local treatment or application of any wound covering. Wound cleansers are solutions used to remove urine, feces, debris, necrotic or foreign matter, and exudate from the wound or surrounding skin. Cleansers often hold antimicrobial and deodorizing properties. In addition to wound cleansers, wound irrigation or hydrotherapy might be indicated to reduce bacterial load within a wound. Hydrotherapy, sometimes known as whirlpool, provides either a selective or non-selective mechanical debriding process to cleanse wounds with thick exudate, necrotic slough or eschar. This wound cleansing process is thought to be most effective for pressure ulcers, venous-related ulcerations, tunneling wounds, infected surgical wounds, contaminated wounds, burns, and others possessing heavy bacterial load. The challenge to caregivers and the obese patient involves transportation of a heavy, unstable patient

around water, narrow lifts, and limited staff. In the outpatient wound or hydrotherapy areas, there must be adequate equipment and preparation to manage the patient. Regardless of the process selected, the objective is to reduce the bacterial load without damaging the surrounding tissue or the wound bed.

## LOCAL TREATMENT: WOUND COVERINGS

There are literally hundreds of categories of wound coverings, and within each category there are a number of options manufactured by the numerous vendors interested in providing wound care products. Although this means that there are an almost limitless number of options available to clinicians, it also means that selecting an intervention can be overwhelming. Included here are the more common and widely used local treatments, although many more exist and will exist as our population ages, the prevalence of obesity increases, and the demand for appropriate wound care modalities grows.

Transparent film dressings are impermeable to liquid, water, and bacteria, but permeable to moisture vapor and atmospheric gases. Because of the transparent nature of these products, they more

fully allow for visualization of the wound bed. Transparent dressings are used as a primary or secondary covering, and are designed to manage partial-thickness wounds with little to no drainage, burns, lacerations, and abrasions. Care should be taken when removing this category of dressing from fragile skin. If the obese patient has taken steroid-type medications for pulmonary problems, a secondary fragility of the skin may develop. Caution must be taken in this case. Skin tears due to removal of the transparent dressing can be very painful, and should be avoided even if it means not using this modality for those at-risk patients.

Hydrogels are formulations of water, polymers, and other ingredients that lack shape. They are designed to provide moisture to an otherwise dry wound, therefore maintaining a moist healing environment. This wound product may be in gel form or impregnated into a dressing sheet. It is indicated for partial- and full-thickness wounds, including necrotic wounds, minor burns, and radiation tissue damage.

Hydrocolloids are usually used as a wafer-type product, composed of gelatin, pectin, carboxymethylcellulose, or other combination. The adhesive wafer is placed over the wound surface and acts to absorb fluid and provide a moist environment. This product is thought to work well over contoured areas because it is moldable to irregular skin surfaces, including skin folds. It is indicated for partial-thickness wounds without necrotic material. And if used with a wound filler, hydrocolloids can also be used to manage full-thickness wounds.

Wound fillers are available as beads, creams, foams, gels, ointments, pads, pastes, pillows, powders, strands, ropes, and other compositions. They are categorically non-adherent and may or may not hold antimicrobial properties. Fillers are placed within a wound cavity, and function to fill dead space and ensure a moist wound bed while managing excess exudate. They require use of a secondary dressing, and in the obese patient the secondary dressing must be able to contour any irregular areas, including folds. Wound fillers are indicated for partial- and full-thickness wounds, draining wounds, and wound that otherwise would require packing. Wound fillers can be useful in managing certain kinds of infected wounds.

Silver-type technology is a category of wound covering that delivers the antimicrobial effects of silver while maintaining a moist environment. Small amounts of silver are delivered to the wound surface over an extended period of time. This type of wound covering is indicated to help reduce the risk of infection in partial- and full-thickness wounds or surgical incisions. This technology is available on a number of different wound coverings, such as transparent films, island dressings, and nonadherent barriers.

Biguanides, like the silver products, offer a topical microbial quality. However, this important class of cationic surface-active antimicrobial agent is thought to resist bacterial colonization within the dressing and reduce bacterial penetration through the dressing. Because of the broad-spectrum effectiveness of this agent, it provides protection against gram-negative, gram-positive, and fungi/yeast organisms, including methicillin-resistant *Staphylococcus aureus* (MRSA) and vancomycin-resistant enterococci (VRE). The biguanide product is impregnated into gauze-type products.

Debriding agents, derived from enzymes or chemicals, are not considered wound dressings; instead they are compounds, which digest necrotic material within acute or chronic wounds. This category of wound product is indicated for debridement of necrotic tissue in pressure ulcers, burns, postoperative wounds, traumatic wounds, or infectious wounds. Debriding agents have been used successfully on necrotic, abdominal blisters; however, determining the etiology of the blisters may serve the greatest good.

Antimicrobials are described as those agents found in creams, ointments, lotions, or sprays that are designed to be applied topically to wounds wherein the goal is to reduce the level of bacterial invasion, therefore reducing odor and other predictable sequelae.

Growth factors are not wound coverings but provide an important topical adjunct in managing wounds that meet certain criteria. Polypeptides are a naturally occurring substance in the human body. These proteins are an important piece in the wound healing puzzle. Research suggests that growth factors stimulate cell growth and migration, and are most effective in the presence of a comprehensive wound management effort. As with all specialized wound dressings and treatment methods, certain criteria must be met. This is especially true with growth factors. It is in the best interest of the patient for the clinician to fully understand the inclusion criteria for this category of product, as it is clearly not indicated for all types of wounds.

## SUMMARY

Any disruption in the skin surface can be costly both emotionally and economically. Care of the obese patient with a wound can be challenging because of comorbidities, immobility, challenges of assessment, and the very diverse assortment of local and systemic treatments available to caregivers. Despite education, clinical skills, and motivation, it can be very difficult for the wound care clinician to deliver safe, effective skin and wound care for the obese patient. Clinicians across the country are looking with an element of frustration at creative strategies to achieve this goal. Policies and procedures typically assist in providing care for complex costly patient groups by employing a standardized method of delivering care based on specific criteria.[15]

The value of an interdisciplinary team cannot be overlooked. The physician, pharmacist, clinical nurse specialist, physical therapist, infection control practitioner, and patient need to have voices in managing complex wounds.

Some centers include vendor input because vendors have resources that may be helpful in better understanding specific qualities of more complex products.

Research is increasingly suggesting that wound develop and wound healing is delayed because of issues with obesity, and failure to recognize the need to address the complex nature of wounds. This is why it is increasingly important to nurture collaborative relationships.

## REFERENCES

1. Gallagher SM. Obesity and the skin care in the critical care area. *Crit Care Nursing* Q. 2002;25(1):69–75.
2. Yeast infections. Available at: www.healthmatters.ca/zellers/ health/PatientInfo.asp?DiseaseNa me=yeast+infections. Access date: April, 2004.
3. Gallagher S. Meeting the needs of the obese patient. *Am J Nurs* 1996;(8suppl):1–14.
4. Engel BT, Burgio KL, Matthews KA. Prevalence incidence and correlates of urinary incontinence in healthy middle aged women. *J Urol* 1991;46(5):1255–9.
5. Steers WD, Suratt PM. Sleep apnea as a cause of daytime and nocturnal enuresis. *Lancet* 1997;349(9069):1604.
6. Foot symptoms. Available at: ale-gent.iqhealth.com//atoz/foot/ symptoms.htm. Access date: April, 2004
5. Gallagher S. Taking the weight off. *Nursing* 2004;34(4):58–64.
6. Davidson J, Callery C. Care of the obesity surgery patient requiring immediate level care or intensive care. *Obesity Surgery* 2001;11:93–7.
7. Gallagher SM. Caring for obese patients. *Nursing 98* 1998;98(3):32HN1–32HN5.
8. Lasater Erhard M. The effect of

patient position of arterial oxygen saturation. *Crit Care Nurs Q* 1995;15:31–6.
9. Gallagher S, Gates J. Obesity, panniculitis, panniculectomy, and wound care: Understanding the challenges. *J WOCN* 2003;30:334–41.
10. Gallagher SM. Obesity and the skin care in the critical care area. *Crit Care Nurs Q* 2002;25(1):69–75.
11. Shinohara E, Kihara S, Yamashita S, et al. Visceral fat accumulation as an important risk factor for obstructive sleep apnea syndrome in obese subjects. *J Intern Med* 1997;241:11–18.
12. Gallagher SM. Caring for obese patients. *Nursing 98* 1998;98(3):32HN1–32HN5.
13. Gallagher S, Langlois C, Spacht D, et al. Preplanning with protocols for skin and wound care among obese patients. *Adv Skin Wound Care* 2004;17(8):436–43.
14. Loehne HB. Pulsatile lavage with concurrent suction. In: Sussman C. *Wound Care: A Collaborative Practice Manual for Physical Therapists and Nurses.* Gaithersburg, MD: Aspen Publishers, 2001
15. National Task Force on the Prevention and Treatment of Obesity. Medical care for obese patients: Advise for healthcare professionals. *Am Fam Phys* 2002;65:81–8.

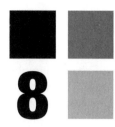

**8**

# Lymphedema and Lipedema

Lymphedema, a disorder of the lymphatic system, affects at least three million Americans.[1] The lymphatic system plays a role in both immune function and circulation. The system comprises lymphatic vessels located just under the skin and lymph nodes that are located in areas around the neck, axilla, and groin. As the vessels transport fluid away from the tissues, waste products, bacteria, and large protein molecules are collected. The fluid is carried to the lymph nodes where the water products are degraded and eliminated, while the remaining protein-rich fluid is transported to the heart and back into circulation.

Symptoms emerge because of the abnormal accumulation of protein rich lymphatic fluid that collects in the interstitial tissue and causes swelling, most often in the arm and/or legs, and occasionally in other parts of the body. This occurs when the normal lymphatic channels are disrupted. When the disruption becomes profound, the lymphatic fluid exceeds the lymphatic transport capacity, leading to lymphedema.

Primary lymphedema is caused by malformations of the lymphatic system, such as when lymphatic vessels are missing or impaired. This can affect any or all parts of the body and is congenital in nature. On the other hand, secondary lymphedema, sometimes referred to as acquired lymphedema, might occur when lymphatic vessels are damaged or lymph nodes are removed. The lymphatic vessels can become damaged as a result of trauma, surgery, radiation, severe chronic venous insufficiency, morbid obesity, or infection.

Without appropriate intervention, protein-rich fluid causes the tissue channels to increase in size and number. This also contributes to a reduction in the oxygen availability in the transport system, which interferes with wound healing and provides for a culture medium for bacteria. This increased bacterial load can result in lymphangitis. When this continues unchecked, the protein-rich fluid continues to accumulate, leading to increased swelling and fibrotic tissue. Untreated lymphedema can lead to a decrease or loss of functioning of the limb, skin breakdown, or chronic infections (See: Untreated Lymphedema).

**CASE REPORT**

**W**illiam, a 450-pound, 52-year-old man, seen in the outpatient wound care center recurrently, suffered from extensive swelling of his lower legs. Although he responded well to manual lymphatic drainage therapy, he had difficulty with both bandaging and graduated compression garments because they simply did not fit properly on his unusually shaped lower leg. This situation is not unusual among very obese patients whose legs are configured like an inverted bottle. Extra padding has been helpful for some patients. In bandaging, a panty girdle or bike shorts can help to keep garments in place, a stockinette can help to decrease slippage if it is long enough at the top to fold over the bandages several inches and pulled up smoothly so that you are not bandaging over wrinkles. Consider use of paper tape on each layer of bandages, especially around the knee, to keep the layers from separating and slipping. Some patients wear snug leggings or stretch pants over the bandages to decrease the friction of the bandages rubbing together between the thighs. Consider Circaid by Beiersdorf-JOBST or compression bandages by Conco.

**STAGES OF LYMPHEDEMA[6]**

- **Stage 1 is spontaneously reversible with pitting edema. Upon waking in the morning, the affected area is normal or almost normal in size.**
- **Stage 2 is spontaneously irreversible; the tissue is spongy in consistency, and nonpitting, fibrotic changes begin.**
- **Stage 3, referred to as lymphostatic elephantiasis, presents as very large extremities with fibrotic tissue. It is unresponsive to intervention. The area becomes a medium for bacterial invasion and subsequent lymphangitis.**

## RISK FACTORS

According to the World Health Organization (UN/WHO), approximately 250 million people acquire lymphedema every year. The most common etiology is the mosquito-born microfilia parasitic infection found in the tropics. However, in industrialized nations, the onset of lymphedema is most commonly associated with complications following cancer treatment. Women are particularly a risk for lymphedema to the arms following surgery or radiation for breast cancer and the legs following treatment for cervical or uterine cancer. Men are at risk of developing lymphedema in

## AIRLINE TRAVEL

**W**hen flying, the decrease in cabin pressure and the dependent position of the lower legs predisposes the patient to swelling due to both the lymphatic and circulatory systems. Listen to Carolyn's thoughts: "I recently gained a significant amount of weight, and even though I have a very high body mass index (BMI), I can still fit in an airline seat. The last time that I flew, I developed an incredible feeling of heaviness in my legs and hips. The heaviness decreases during the night, and resolved some in the morning, but by mid-morning the swelling and heaviness have returned and were very uncomfortable." Without additional information, it is difficult to point to Carolyn's exact issue; however, most would agree that if a thorough physical revealed lymphedema there are options for Carolyn. In the event that Carolyn flew frequently, she would be best served by employing manual lymph drainage, including long-term use of graduated compression garments.

their legs following surgery for prostrate or testicular cancer. Both men and women are at risk following treatment for malignant melanoma or any other surgery or radiation affecting the lymph nodes or requiring lymph node dissection. For example, 50 to 70 percent of patients having axillary lymph node dissection develop lymphedema. It is estimated 1 to 2 million breast cancer survivors are alive today, and 400,000 of them cope daily with disfigurement.

## UNDERSTANDING LYMPHEDEMA

The lymphatic system provides a filtering system for the entire body. Lymph nodes are placed strategically throughout the body and where they serve as filtering

stations for lymphatic fluid. These vessels lead to and from the nodes and are located superficially as well as deep within the tissue and vary in size. Any damage or occlusion to the lymphatic structure can lead to interruption in lymphatic flow and consequently lymphatic accumulation and congestion, the clinical manifestation of lymphedema.[2] Lymphedema should not be confused with edema, which results from venous insufficiency and is not lymphedema. However, untreated venous insufficiency can progress into a combined venous/lymphatic disorder, which is treated in ways similar to treatment of lymphedema. Also, lipedema must be differentiated from lymphedema; however, treatment overlap can occur in this condition as well.

## UNDERSTANDING LIPEDEMA

Lipedema is characterized by a bilateral, symmetrical increase in stored fat, which usually affects the hips, buttocks, and thighs. The fibers in the fatty tissue multiply and thicken, which also give rise to an increase in connective tissue pressure and eventually hardening of the collagen fibers. There is a feeling of heaviness and, unlike lymphedema, this type of edema is painful in advanced stages and the legs bruise easily. Patients with lipedema are not usually at risk for infections as those with lymphedema. Although the swelling can be extensive, it seldom involves the feet. Interestingly enough, the person's torso may be very thin.

Lipedema often develops at the time of puberty, can be familial, and affects women. This hormonally driven condition can be controlled as long the woman remains thin and active. Unfortunately, once the patient begins to gain weight, the condition progresses rapidly. Many women with lipedema become morbidly obese because of weight gain coupled with difficulty comfortably achieving an adequate level of activity.[3]

In fact, one of the primary problems with lipedema is that it leads to inactivity.

**UNTREATED LYMPHEDEMA CAN LEAD TO:**

- Increased limb swelling
- Reduced range of motion
- Permanent disfigurement
- Limb heaviness
- Fungal infection
- Invasive biological infections
- Recurrent lymphangitis
- Lymphadenitis
- Bacteremia
- Lymphatic destruction
- Thrombosis lymphatica
- Hyperkeratosis
- Fissuring
- Cellulitis
- Reduction of lymphatic or vascular circulation
- Chronic ulceration
- Tissue necrosis
- Gangrene
- Amputation

**CONTRAINDICATIONS TO COMPLEX DECONGESTIVE THERAPY**

- Swelling of unknown origin
- Recurrent tumor or disease
- Lymphangitis
- Suspect deep vein thrombosis
- Unexplained pain
- Unmonitored congestive heart failure

obesity. Others fail to recognize the difference between cellulite and lipedema. Panniculopathia edematicosclerotica, often referred to as simply cellulite, is a related but different condition, which occurs in young women and causes changes in the subcutaneous tissues of the thighs, buttocks, and hips. Yet some patients are affected by lipolymphedema, a condition in which lymphedema occurs as a secondary effect of lipedema. If the patient becomes overweight, the excess fatty tissue compresses the superficial lymphatic vessels, interfering with normal function of the lymphatic system.

Many patients who have lipedema become overweight and encounter difficulty losing weight. There are several types of exercise that are best avoided, such as high impact or intense, repetitive activities. Swimming, walking, and core strengthening are some options. To compound issues with weight, lipedema interferes with metabolism of certain fats. Long chain fatty acids are absorbed by the lacteals, which are part of the lymphatic system in the small intestine, thus absorbed into the lymphatic system. Once digested, long chain fatty acids go on to be stored in adipose tissue to be used

Physical fatigue can develop with a corresponding need for rest. Women with lipedema are likely to gain weight for a number of reasons. For example, many women avoid sports because they feel tired much of the time. It becomes difficult to climb stairs, wear regular clothing, or even walk. Others fail to engage in vigorous activity because they are embarrassed by the appearance of

their body. Each of these factors work together to contribute to progressive weakness, additional weight gain, compulsive eating, increased reclusivity, and further development of lipedema.

Another problem is the widespread misunderstanding of lipedema. Clinicians tend to misunderstand lipedema and its role with lymphedema. Lipedema is often confused with morbid

later. There is belief that medium fatty acids (MCT) in the diet can help to alleviate the problem. Medium chain fatty acids bypass the intestines and are absorbed by the liver. They are easily absorbed and unlike other fats, they put little strain on the digestive system and provide a quick source of energy. Because medium chain fatty acids are digested and absorbed quickly with minimal effort, there is less strain on the pancreas, liver, and the digestive system. Pure virgin cold pressed coconut oil is a medium fatty acid. Caprylic acid is a medium chain fatty acid derived from coconut oil found to exhibit antifungal properties on contact with the fungus. Once absorbed, caprylic acid is no longer antifungal but is then metabolized to produce energy. Caprylic acid is produced in the body in small amounts and is a natural component of coconut oil, palm nut oil, butterfat, and other vegetable and animal sources. It is synthesized from caprylic alcohol, sometimes referred to as octanol, and is found in coconut oil. A diet high in vegetables, fish, fruits, whole grains, and omega fatty acids is advised. The patient should avoid refined carbohydrates and sugar, as well as limit intake of sodium.

## LYMPHEDEMA, LIPEDEMA, OR VENOUS DISEASE?

Elizabeth is a 52-year-old woman who is not sure if she has lymphedema, lipedema, venous disease, edema, or all of the above. Despite her diagnosis of lymphedema secondary to deep vein thrombus, several clinicians have suggested the condition may be more complicated than originally thought. Clinically her symptoms are as follows: clear yellow fluid draining from several small open areas, light brownish discoloration of the lower leg, aching pain, deep hardened folds on both ankles, and papillomas on the skin-all typical of phlebo-lymphostatic edema. Deep vein thrombus (DVT) causes significant damage to the deep veins, which eventually leads to edema. The lymphatic system is designed to help maintain this by transporting the excess fluid from the area. If left untreated, venous edema will overwhelm the lymphatic vessels and consequently tax the local lymphatic system causing it too to become diseased. This downward spiral can be accelerated by infections, such as phlebitis and cellulitis, dependent position, activity, and obesity. The brownish discoloration is called hemosiderin staining and is a vein disease problem. It often indicates very poor blood circulation and high pressure in the area of discoloration. Wounds develop due to poor cellular nutrition and delayed healing following longstanding swelling and minor injury. In regard to the lymphedema component, hardening of the tissues, thick wart-like skin patches, and or square toes and folds are classic signs that the lymphatic system has failed. Treatment for combined diagnoses is the same as for pure lymphedema. Complete decongestive therapy (CDT) can be highly successful when used in conjunction with weight and stress management, exercise, and nutrition long term.

## OBESITY AND LYMPHEDEMA

Obesity stresses the delicate lymphatic vessels, and serves as a significant risk factor in lymphedema. If untreated, lymphedema leads to tissue breakdown, limited motion, and recurrent cellulitis. Lymphedema may be precipitated or made worse by cellulitis, and cellulitis is more difficult to treat in the presence of lymphedema.

## CLINICAL IMPLICATIONS

Once a definitive diagnosis is made and the client understands the chronicity of lymphatic challenges, certain treatment procedures can begin. Complete decongestive therapy (CDT) is a safe, reliable, and noninvasive technique, and is considered the gold standard for care. CDT is a four-step process comprising manual lymph drainage (MLD); graduated compression garments; therapeutic exercise; and scrupulous skin care.

CDT works in two steps. The first step includes strategies to move the lymphatic fluid out of the affected region and reduce the swelling using MLD techniques and compression bandaging. MLD is a gentle hands-on technique that stimulates the activity of the lymphatic vessels and manually moves lymphatic fluid. Applied correctly, a series of MLD treatments will generally decrease the volume of the affected extremity to normal or near normal size. Ideally these treatments are done daily, five days a week for 2 to 4 weeks, depending on the severity. Bandages are applied during this time to retain the achieved reduction. Once the swelling is reduced, the patient is fitted with a graduated compression garment. This marks the second phase.

The compression garment is essential to maintain the success of MLD because the vessels must work much harder to accomplish the task of lymphatic return. In other words, the lymphatic system needs external support. Graduated compression garments are necessary to maintain the reduced limb and are designed to replace bandages that were used earlier in the treatment process. The compression garments are worn during the day. Wearing a compression garment provides necessary external support to the extent that it provides assistance to lymphatic drainage. Compression garments can be especially helpful when the client engages in repetitive motion, such as housecleaning, gardening, and some forms of physical activity or exercise. The objective of the graduated compression garment is to reduce swelling and prevent reaccumulation of lymphatic fluid in the area. In addition to compression garments, meticulous skin care, self manual lymphatic drainage, and therapeutic exercise will promote success.

In the presence of lipedema, chronic venous insufficiency, or lymphedema, the skin is usually dry and fissures easily, creating a susceptibility to cellulitis and other types of infection. Encourage the patient to avoid tight or restrictive clothing that impairs circulation or causes irritation, skin scratches, or swelling. Shoes with low heels are recommended, especially if lower leg edema exists. Jewelry, such as watches, anklets, bracelets, or finger or toe

**SUPPLIERS**

**Bandages Direct**
**866-99-LYMPH**

**Bandages Plus Inc**
**800-770-1032**

**Compression Management Services, Inc.**
**877-267-4415**

**Healthy Legs**
**Healthylegs.com**

**Jobst Hosiery Direct**
**SupportHoseStore.com**

**JUZO**
**888-255-1300**

**LymphaCare Lymphedema Product and Reimbursement Specialists**
**888-854-2228**

**Remarx Medical Services**
**www.remarxservices.com**

**TUNU**
**www.tunu.com**

**CONSIDERING REIMBURSEMENT**

**K**eep in mind that a compression garment is not an article of clothing, but a prosthetic device that replaces pressure that is lost by missing or damaged lymphatics. Compression garments help to maintain fluid balance in a limb. Many insurance carriers understand the language of prosthetics.

rings, should not fit tightly or rub against the skin surface. Keep skin protected by using a mild cleanser and lotion that are free of alcohol or fragrances daily. Explain to the patient that bath water should be warm but not hot. Avoid irritating cosmetics, detergents, deodorants, or perfumes. Use sunblock and insect repellent regularly. The area should be inspected daily for discoloration, changes in temperature, texture variation, or pain. Any of these together or separately should be reported to the primary care provider.

A skilled therapist may recommend activities that are suited to the client's unique needs, abilities, and resources. An appropriate program that assists the muscular system in moving lymphatic fluid out of the affected area is one strategy. It is important to avoid injury and overexertion in the affected area, with low or no-impact activities being the best. Increased weight complicates lymphedema. Maintain a balanced diet that includes a lot of fruits, vegetables, whole grains, and proteins. Encourage patients to avoid excessive fatty foods, sweets, alcohol, and salt. Drink plenty of water and unsweetened beverages. Moderate exercise, such as swimming, walking, biking, and core strengthening are some options. High impact sports, heavy weight lifting, and aggressive contact activities should be avoided.

Use of diuretics should be considered carefully, as some literature cautions against their use. For example, diuretics will initially decrease the water content and reduce swelling, but the protein molecules remain in the tissues and swelling will recur as soon as the drug loses its effectiveness.

## LOWER LEG INFECTION

Cellulitis (infection) is a common complication among patients with lymphedema because of changes in the skin function. The skin's acid film of protection is destroyed in edematous tissue and the immunity in the skin is lowered. Cellulitis is an infection of the dermis and subcutaneous tissue and is usually caused by streptococcus or staphylococcus organisms. It is characterized by warmth, edema, erythema, and advancing borders. Patients clinically may develop fevers and elevated white blood cell counts that may progress to local tissue death and systemic infection. Cellulitis can develop in seemingly healthy skin, but usually develops in the presence of a break in the skin. Hygiene, friction to the skin surface, and the inability to examine and clean the lower extremity places the patient at risk. Cellulitis usually results in blistering of the epidermis, and superficial necrosis might be present. The extent of the injury can range from acute erythema, with or without blisters, to extensive epidermal necrosis with exudate.

In the presence of obesity, the adipose tissue is thicker in the lower extremity. When ulcers develop they can be difficult to treat. Itching and soreness are not unusual, and symptoms are often disregarded until pain, swelling, and fever make treatment essential. Patients should be encouraged to access care in a timely and appropriate manner.

Early assessment and intervention is imperative, as cellulitis can further aggravate lymphedema. Elevated intraabdominal pressure is associated with poor circulation, and thus impaired circulation can delay response to treatment should the patient develop cellulitis.

Treatment is aimed at resolving the acute infection and preventing recurrent episodes of cellulitis. The mainstay of treatment is antibiotic therapy. Antibiotics are often required intravenously in the initial stages of infection and can be changed to oral once the infection begins to resolve.[4] Empirical treatment with a penicillinase-resistant penicillin, first generation cephalosporin, amoxicillin-clavulanate macrolide, or fluoroquinolone is appropriate.[5] A 4 to 6 week course of treatment may be necessary because of impaired circulation to the area.

## CONCLUSION

Lymphedema is a chronic condition that must be managed every day. Ongoing therapy can be taxing for patients, and lifelong changes must be made. The role of the clinician is to support the patient, not only by managing the lymphedema and related physical issues, but addressing the emotional, social, and spiritual aspects of care.

## REFERENCES

1.  What is lymphedema? Available at: www.remarxservices.com. Access date: June 2005.
2.  Lymphedema: System interrupted. Available at: www.lymphdoc.com . Access date: June 2005.
3.  Lipedema. Available at: lymphedema.com/lipedema.htm. Access date: June 2005.
4.  Baxter H, McGregor F. Understanding and managing cellulitis. *Nsg Standard* 2001;15(44):50–5.
5.  Sulberg D, Penrod M, Blatny R. Common bacterial skin infections *Am Fam Phys* 2002:66(1):119–24.
6.  Symptoms of lymphedema. Available at: www.lymphnet.org/whatis.html. Access date: June 2005.

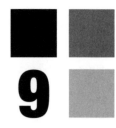

**9**

# Panniculectomy

**P**anniculectomy surgery becomes necessary for many patients who have had massive weight loss due to successful bariatric weight loss surgery.[1] Bariatric weight loss surgery is one of the fastest growing specialties in America; therefore, clinicians can expect to care for increasing numbers of patients who require this reconstructive procedure.

Panniculectomy, by definition, is the surgical removal of an abdominal panniculus, commonly referred to as an abdominal apron. The panniculus is the redundant layer of fatty tissue at the lowest portion of the abdominal wall. This abnormal deposit of fatty tissue aggravates various complications associated with obesity.

This chapter will review the five grades of panniculus and the physical challenges associated with surgically removing 100 pounds or more of redundant skin, fat, muscle and vasculature. Documentation for reimbursement, postoperative care, and recent theories pertaining to surgical removal of large amounts of adipose tissue are also described. The common, predictable, and costly complications, such as pain, immobility, and skin injury, are reviewed.

## BARIATRIC WEIGHT LOSS SURGERY (BWLS)

Because of the ongoing concerns pertaining to postoperative problems with the pannus, some surgeons have opted to remove the panniculus at the time of initial weight loss surgery. Other surgeons prefer to wait 12 to 24 months until the patient has lost most of the weight that will be lost. Each technique holds advantages and disadvantages, and the choice as to one or the other is largely decided between the patient and his or her surgeon(s).

Regardless, increasing numbers of patients are losing very large amounts of excess weight due to improved bariatric surgical techniques. While this allows the patients to take advantage of the physical, social, psychological, and economic benefits of bariatric surgery, they are often left with extra skin, abnormal fat deposits, and bodily deformities. These deformities could lead to functional, psychosocial, and medical comorbidities. These comorbidities can adversely affect the overall outcome of an otherwise successful bariatric surgery. In order to fully benefit from successful weight loss, additional surgical correction may be required. In many cases, panniculectomy surgery becomes essential fol-

---

**TOTAL BODY LIFT**

Irene Orr, interviewed on KNBC-4 television, reports losing 205 pounds, which left her with a considerable amount of loose skin. Like Orr, more patients are opting for the total body lift because panniculectomy was not enough. Dr. Milton Owens describes the total body lift as a procedure to remove 7 to 25 pounds of loose skin by surgically removing skin from the thighs, buttocks, and abdomen. Owens and Orr concur that significant pain is associated with the procedure; however, Orr was back to work six weeks after the surgery. To view the interviews, visit www.coastalobesity.com/News.htm.

---

lowing bariatric weight loss surgery.[2–9]

## PANNICULECTOMY

Panniculectomy surgery simply refers to removal of the abdominal pannus. However, in addition to panniculectomy, some surgeons combine reconstructive abdominoplasty with panniculectomy surgery. The surgery may also include suction lipoplasty to improve the reconstructed abdominal wall contour as well as umbilical or ventral hernia repair.[10]

The panniculectomy incision extends from the sternoxiphoid process to the pubic bone. There it meets a second horizontal incision just above the pubic area to form what looks like an inverted letter "T." In order to create this "T," the surgeon frees up fat and skin from the anterior abdomen. At that point, a large triangularly shaped area of loose skin and excess fat is carefully removed. The remaining tissue is then attached to the anterior abdom-

inal wall and to itself. A number of procedures can be completed at the same time, such as exploratory laparotomy, revision of the primary surgery, repair of abdominal wall/ventral hernia, or others.[10]

## SURGICAL EXPERIENCE

In comparing BWLS and panniculectomy surgery, the latter may be a more involved procedure for some patients. However, following significant weight loss, the risks associated with panniculectomy surgery are reduced. But the complex nature of this procedure should alert clinicians and patients to the need for vigilant care.

The preoperative period for the morbidly obese patient consists of both physical and emotional preparation. Because of the risks for pulmonary problems, the very overweight patient will need to pay special attention to comprehensive preoperative teaching, which includes breathing and coughing instructions and appropriate

**PANNUS ASSESSMENT TOOL GRADING SYSTEM**

- Grade 1—covers the pubic hairline but not the entire mons pubis
- Grade 2—extends to cover the entire mons pubis
- Grade 3—extends to cover the upper thigh
- Grade 4—extends to mid thigh
- Grade 5—extends to the knee and beyond

**ABDOMINAL PANNICULUS AND ASSOCIATED COMORBIDITIES ICD9CM CODES**

| | |
|---|---|
| • Abdominal mass, diffuse | 789.3 |
| • Hypertrophic or atrophic skin | 701.6 |
| • Panniculitis | 729.39 |
| • Panniculitis affecting back | 724.8 |
| • Skin abscess, abdominal wall | 682.2 |
| • Hernia | 553.0 |
| • Dermatitis | 692.9 |

leg exercises.[2] Breathing and coughing exercises are especially important to prevent atelectasis and congestion that can result from shallow respirations as a result of incisional pain, depressive analgesia, inactivity, and obesity itself.[3] Demonstrations of deep breathing and coughing exercises should include splinting the involved surgical area and use of the incentive spirometer. Patients need to be reminded that gentle splinting will not interfere with the abdominal incisions.

Obesity is a major risk factor for postoperative thrombophlebitis, deep vein thrombosis, and pulmonary embolism. This may be due to an elevated hemoglobin and hematocrit, which occurs in the presence of obesity hypoventilation syndrome (OHS). Increased red cell production is the body's natural response to hypercapnia and many obese patients experience this due to OHS and other respiratory issues.[4]

Successful preoperative preparation includes identifying the patient's family or other support person. This person will be instrumental in postoperative care and must be included in teaching, especially if the patient has a prolonged hospitalization, visual barriers in caring for the incision, or generalized weakness. An atmosphere of understanding, cooperation, and trust ensure a smoother postoperative course for the patient.

Intraoperative care is highly specialized and, among other goals, ensures patient safety and while attending to prevention of caregiver injury. Generally, two nurses are required at surgical procedures: a scrub nurse and a circulating nurse. In caring for larger patients, some institutions provide a third nurse, especially at the beginning of the procedure. The third nurse may be necessary for positioning. A task as simple as placing a catheter can be technically difficult, and an unnecessary embarrassment to the patient, so often the catheter is placed once the patient has been properly sedated or anesthetized.[5]

Another intervention of concern that has particular interest in caring for larger patients is the surgical scrub or preparation of the skin surface. The nurse must ensure that all areas are clean and painted vigorously. This can be especially difficult in the presence of deep skin folds and irregular contours. Excess skin cleansers should not be left to pool within skin folds as this can lead to irritation and subsequent breakdown in skin integrity. The third nurse is helpful to the circulation nurse in achieving this task.

Once the surgery is completed, a larger gown must be readily available, eliminating embarrassment to the patient at the last minute. Extra personnel may be required to place the patient onto a gurney, or perhaps an oversized bed that will go with the patient to his or her room once recovery is accomplished. Recovery staff needs to be notified that they will be receiving a larger patient, which allows for any necessary preplanning.

Preplanning helps prevent last minute scrambling to find tools essential for post-operative assessment. Standard sized equipment, such as a blood pressure cuff, may be insufficient to accomplish simple assessment. The patient may be discharged from the recovery room to either the intensive care unit or a general medical surgery unit, depending on medical assessment or hospital policy. It best serves the clinical needs of the patient and the safety needs of caregivers to have a plan for

care in place prior to admission.[6]

In the acute setting, patients can experience complications related to immobility and physical dependence. Some patients will fail to progress postoperatively either because of surgical complications or a critical condition. Clinicians need to be familiar with common obesity-related complications, and modify patient care plans and clinical intervention to address or prevent them.

Although the patient is often awake and alert shortly after surgery, extra personnel are required to transfer the patient to the appropriate postoperative unit as lateral transfers are a growing threat to caregiver safety. Neck and shoulder pain are fast becoming as prevalent as back injury as an adverse

outcome of moving dependent patients. A hover-type product may ensure a safe transfer while protecting the caregiver from injury.

A number of conditions affect the patient's postoperative course. Early mobilization is critical in the recovery period. Many larger patients are able to turn, ambulate, and transfer soon after surgery, while others may have difficulty because of pain or sedation.[7] As a member of the interdisciplinary team, the physical therapist can assess the strength, endurance, and equipment needs of the patient. Patients who weigh more than 300 pounds generally require some level of special accommodation. Many times the only special accommodation needed is a bed that is wide enough for the patient to turn independently, a walker to support his or her weight for the first few postoperative days, and an overhead trapeze to help the patient reposition him or herself. These three items are thought to help the patient maintain strength and independence. And clinicians report that independent patients who have adequate supportive equipment are less likely to injure themselves or caregivers during that early postoperative period.[8]

Routine monitoring of vital signs and physiologic progress requiring careful documentation include blood pressure, pulse, quality and number of respirations per minute, temperature, coughing, and deep breathing. Physical conditions can change quickly; therefore, a baseline assessment with frequent, regular monitoring can prevent delays in care. Sequential compression devices to accommodate the larger leg are available, and to that extent foot "squeezers" are useful in that they usually better accommodate the larger patient.

Obese immobile patients often present with atypical pressure ulcers. Pressure within skin folds can be sufficient to cause skin breakdown. Tubes and catheters can burrow into skin folds, further eroding the skin surface. Pressure from side rails and arm rests not designed to accommodate a larger person can cause pressure ulcers on the patient's hips. This atypical skin breakdown can be minimized with appropriate assessment and timely, appropriate intervention.[9]

Wound healing can be problematic in some obese patients. Blood supply to fatty tissue may be insufficient to provide an adequate amount of oxygen and nutrients. This can lead to wound dehiscence, evisceration, or infection delays in healing. Wound healing may also be delayed if the patient has a diet that lacks essential vitamins and nutrients. Infection can be a problem because many morbidly obese patients have asso-

ciated medical problems, particularly type 2 diabetes mellitus. In fact, 80 percent of noninsulin dependent diabetics are obese.[10] This contributes to delayed wound healing.

Although hematoma formation rarely occurs, seroma formation is a common problem.[11] Drains are routinely placed after surgery to prevent seroma formation. It is important to watch for clotting of the drains, unintentional removal of the drains by the patient, or pressure sufficient to occlude flow from the drains simply because the drain became lodged in a skin fold. Patients frequently are discharged to home with drains in place. Patients or their caregivers will need to demonstrate emptying and care of the tubes, as well as a plan in the event the tube clots or falls out.

All skin should be kept clean and dry, especially those in skin folds, where excess moisture and bacteria can accumulate. A clean flannel receiving blanket from the nursery offers one option to prevent the surfaces from coming in contact with one another, thus preventing intertriginous irritation.

In the event wounds develop, it is important to contain any drainage, especially in folds. Clean the area frequently with a non-toxic cleanser, and secure dry dressings to absorb excess moisture. Irregular body contours can present challenges in securing dressings. Flexible

cloth tapes can mold to the contours as necessary to ensure that the dressings are fixed securely to the intended area.

Further, excess body fat also increases the tension at the wound edges.[12] To reduce the occurrence of abdominal wound separation, some clinicians use a surgical binder to support the area. Binders not only provide comfort to the patient, but are designed to minimize the shearing forces between the abdominal wall and abdominal skin.[13] However, if the binder does not fit properly it can lead to skin breakdown or failure to comply with the plan of care. The binder will need to be large enough to comfortably fit the patient: bariatric-sized binders will meet this requirement.

Pain is thought to interfere with mobility and therefore must be considered as part of the care plan. Excess body fat can alter drug absorption, depending on the medication. For example, drugs such as diazepam and carbamazepine are highly soluble in fat and are absorbed mostly in adipose tissue. Dosage of these drugs must be calculated using the patient's actual body weight. Drugs that are absorbed mainly into lean tissue, such as acetaminophen, should be calculated using the patient's ideal body weight.[14] Trying to remember which drugs fall into which category is almost impossible. A

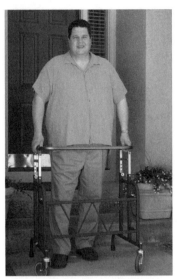

**Early mobilization is critical in the recovery period...Many times the only special accommodation needed is a bed that is wide enough for the patient to turn independently, a walker to support his or her weight for the first few postoperative days, and an overhead trapeze to help the patient reposition him or herself.**

clinical pharmacist can be an important resource to ensure that the drug dose is accurate.[15]

Postoperative care is essential in the beginning of the recovery period for the patient. Early ambulation, appropriate use of specialized equipment, attention to the risks of wound and pulmonary complications, IV access, and pain management all work together to that end.

## DOCUMENTATION FOR REIMBURSEMENT

The abdominal panniculus can weigh as little as five pounds and upward to over 100 pounds. Patients having bariatric weight loss surgery who lose large amounts of weight are often left with a symptomatic pannus. Barriers exist to panniculectomy surgery because of the misconception that the procedure is strictly cosmetic in nature. This misconception arises out of the lay term *tummy tuck*.[16] As some consumers, members of the medical community, and insurance companies have come to realize, obesity is a serious medical problem, which ultimately impacts negatively on quality of life and life span.[1] However, this understanding is not widely held and barriers to appropriate medical intervention continue to exist. Widespread confusion surrounds the challenges of obesity, bariatric weight loss surgery, and panniculectomy. This further complicates the issues of third party reimbursement as decision makers may also misunderstand these complexities.

A large abdominal pannus is associated with cutaneous inflammation, such as panniculitis, cellulitis, intertriginous dermatitis, skin abscesses, gangrene, excoriation, and folliculitis. Other concerns related to the pannus are lymphedema, ambulatory difficulty, toileting trouble, and hygiene problems that can lead to unpleasant odors. Urinary stress incontinence can be aggravated by elevated intra-abdominal pressure along with the extra lower abdominal weight. A large abdominal pannus often poses a barrier to sexual activity. Patients frequently complain of debilitating low back, hip, and extremity pain that interferes with physical activity or simply normal activities of daily living. Clothes fit improperly, and patients report body image concerns. A large abdominal pannus can interfere with respiratory function and can lead to diminished abdominal wall integrity from attenuated fascia and muscles; umbilical and ventral hernias are not uncommon. Abdominal panniculectomy and reconstructive abdominal surgery may be performed to alleviate these associated conditions. However, some third-party payers are reluctant to provide reimbursement, and most patients are unable to afford the procedure without some financial assistance.

Documentation is an important factor in decisions pertaining to reimbursement. An interdisciplinary approach has been the most successful in accomplishing reimbursement. Physicians, physical therapists, pain specialists, occupational therapists and others each offer a unique perspective in building the case for reimbursement.

Indications for panniculectomy require documentation because such documentation both informs decisions and serves as a basis for appeal in the event that the corrective surgery is initially denied.

Third-party payers have been known to refuse payment for abdominal panniculectomy for many reasons, one being a misunderstanding of the nature of the problem. Therefore, it is prudent to document all observed and reported clinical symptoms that are associated with a large abdominal pannus, along with dated photographs.

Some payers require that the pannus extend sufficiently to obscure the pubic area, while in other cases the criteria for coverage has been vague and subjective. Part of the challenge for both clinicians and insurance carriers is that the requirements for reimbursement and the assessment tools to describe the pannus have been equally subjective. For example, previously a pannus has been described as *mild, moderate,* or *severe*. These subjective terms are confusing for clinicians and insurance reviewers. A grading system has recently been introduced that objectively describes five levels based on severity (See Pannus Assessment Tool Grading System). This more objective assessment tool provides for less misunderstanding in that each grade is specifically defined.

ICD-9CM Codes might provide a language recognized by reviewers and could prove help-ful (See Abdominal Panniculus and Associated Comorbidities ICD-9CM Codes). Each ICD code has specific criteria. For a more detailed description of each condition, refer to Characteristics of ICD -9-CM.[12] ICD-9 codes should be attached to diagnostic terms when submitting appeal letters (See Sample Letter of Appeal).

Other insurance reviewers reportedly look for intertrigo or other signs of inflammation under and/or on the pannus. Candidiasis can cause or aggravate intertrigo.[13] Intertrigo, an inflammatory condition of skin folds, is induced or aggravated by heat, moisture, maceration, friction, and lack of air circulation. The condition is frequently exacerbated by infection, which is typically fungal but may also be bacterial or viral. Intertrigo generally affects the axilla, perineum, inframammary creases, and abdominal folds. It is a common complication of obesity and diabetes.[17]

Again, objective assessment, with careful attention to all the clinical signs, best serves the end of reimbursement. Measure open areas, discoloration, and other skin changes. Wounds themselves can present in varying degrees of depth or tissue destruction. Some clinicians describe wounds in terms of a clock face. Wounds may be full or partial thickness. They may be covered with necrotic matter. This necrotic matter may be further described as necrotic eschar or necrotic slough. Reviewers are interested in the amount and nature of wound drainage and whether odor is present. Because of the graphic nature of photographs, it remains essential to provide adjunctive photodocumentation. Patient photos best serve the patient's needs when they include front, side, and under-surface views.

Treatment, including frequency and duration, is important and can be translated into cost figures when necessary. Some patients report considerable time away from work, incurring additional cost consequences.

Although the personnel in the physician's office may submit the request for panniculectomy surgery, without adequate documentation reimbursement may not be granted. The value of an interdisciplinary team cannot be overlooked. The collaborative effort of the team serves to identify the patient's functional limitations due to the symptomatic pannus. For example, the physical and occupational therapists may offer a better understanding of the impact the large pannus has on the patient's ability to engage in activity, or lack thereof. The pain specialist can describe the nature of the patient's pain, and quantitatively report the cost of reasonable pain management. The more comprehensive the team, the more complete the picture. Insurance carriers will need documentation and quantitative data not only in terms of skin and wound problems, but also regarding additional functional limitations.

When all else fails, some patients have asked attorneys who specialize in reimbursement for bariatric needs to assist them in obtaining third party reimbursement.[15] The attorney will typically use the medical record to make the argument for reimbursement. Therefore, the narrative and photographic documentation therein will be critical in pursuing this avenue. A functional assessment by a physical therapist or occupational therapist may help the attorney and insurance carrier determine the extent of physical limitations the pannus poses.

Additionally, the attorney may solicit records of other members of the healthcare team because some patients will suffer with incontinence, breathing difficulties, pain and quality of life challenges, which can also lead to monetary and non-monetary costs. These factors may influence reimbursement decisions.[18]

## SUMMARY

It is important for consumers to realize that weight loss surgery is only a tool to help patients lose weight. Once weight loss is achieved, the patients may continue to struggle with quality of life issues, one of which is a large abdominal pannus. Panniculectomy is performed to remove a massive panniculus, which frequently contributes to functional deficits as well as hygiene and wound care problems. Therefore, panniculectomy surgery is thought to provide the patient with the opportunity to move forward with activities of daily living. Careful, objective documentation that outlines the actual and potential skin and wound complications associated with a large abdominal pannus is critical in influencing reimbursement decisions, which ultimately influences the patient's quality of life.[19]

## REFERENCES

1. Fobi M. Panniculectomy: Time to remove excess abdominal fat. Available at: www.geocities.com/hotsprings/6698/pann.html. Access date: November 2002.
2. French G, Galbraith JL, Dietel M. The nurses' role in bariatric surgery. In: Deitel M. *Surgery for the Morbidly Obese Patient*. Toronto, Canada: FD-Communications, 2000.
3. Crowell DE. Anesthetic management of morbidly obese patient undergoing abdominal surgery: Epidural anesthesia and postoperative epidural anesthesia. In: Deitel M. *Surgery for the Morbidly Obese Patient*. Toronto, Canada: FD-Communications, 2000.
5. Gallagher S. Taking the weight off with bariatric surgery. *Nursing* 2004;34(3)58–64.
6. Gallagher S, Langlois C, Spacht D, et al. Preplanning protocols for skin and wound care in obese patients. *Adv Skin Wound Care* 2004;17(8):436–43.
7. Gallagher SM. Tailoring care for the obese patient. *RN* 1999;62(5):43–50.
8. Gallagher SM. Restructuring the therapeutic environment to promote care and safety for obese patient. *JWOCN* 1999;26:292–7.
9. Gallagher SM. Caring for obese patients. *Nursing 98* 1998;98(3):32HN1–32HN5.
10. Troia C. Promoting positive outcomes in obese patients. *Plas Surg Nurs* 2002;22(1):10–28.
11. Freiberg A. Plastic surgery after massive weight loss. In: Deitel M (ed). *Surgery for the Morbidly Obese Patient*. Toronto, Canada: FD Communications, 2000.
12. Gallagher SM. Morbid obesity: A chronic disease with an impact on wounds and related problems. *Ost Wound Manage* 1997;43(5):18–27.
13. Gallagher S, Gates J. Obesity, panniculitis, panniculectomy, and wound care. *JWOCN* 2003;30(6):334–41.
14. Goodell TT. The obese trauma patient: Treatment strategies. *J Trauma Nurs* 1996;3(2):36.
15. Gallagher SM. Caring for the obese patient. *Nursing 98* 1998;28(3):31hn–33hn.
16. Panniculectomy: More than a tummy tuck. *Nursing* 2004;34(12).
17. Candidiasis of Skin Folds. Available at: www.dermnetnz.org. Access date: January 2005.
18. Seldon S. Intertrigo. Available at: emedicine.com/derm/topic198.htm. Access date: Accessed November 2002.
19. Gallagher S. Panniculectomy, documentation, reimbursement, and the WOC Nurse. *JWOCN* 2003;30(2):72–7.
20. Lindstrom W. So you want your insurance to cover your obesity surgery? Available at: www.obesitylaw.com/insurancearticle.htm. Access date: September 2000.
21. Igwe D, Malgorzata S, Hoil L, et al. Panniculectomy adjuvant to obesity surgery. *Obes Surg* 10:530–9.
22. The International Classification of Diseases. Available at: cedr.lbl.gov/icd9.html. Access date: November 2002.

# Pain Management

**P**ain can interfere with patient mobility and ultimately with patient care for a number physiologic and psychologic reasons. In most cultures, pain serves as a warning that something is wrong. Patients experiencing pain might respond with reluctance to move or participate in activity and mobility. This is especially problematic among obese patients who often encounter numerous threats to immobility. Often reluctance to allow repositioning or to reposition themselves may be misinterpreted as nonadherent or health-defeat-ing behavior that further confounds care and may even threaten the therapeutic relationship.

One of the greatest challenges in healthcare today is to ensure the physical, emotional, and spiritual comfort of our patients. Management of pain is an important factor in patient comfort, and all patients, regardless of size, are entitled to the best pain relief that safely can be achieved. Yet the problem of pain is pervasive, and the myths and misconceptions surrounding the pain experience and the assessment of pain often preclude adequate comfort and quality care. This is especially true among bariatric patients where little evidence-based practice is available to make decisions about patient care and pain management. Pain must be managed adequately because, as research now suggests, unrelieved pain can inhibit the immune system, increase oxygen demand, exacerbate respiratory dysfunction, decrease gastrointestinal motility, and lead to mental confusion. Severe acute pain is a major risk for chronic neuropathic pain.[5] Misconceptions not only affect clinical decisions, but patients may also hold these misunderstandings, further interfering with pain control.

## SPECIAL CHALLENGES TO CONSIDER

In addition to the challenges that all patients face, bariatric patients have additional concerns. More questions than answers arise when dealing with pain in patients whose bodies are a greater percentage of adipose tissue. For example, is the medication of choice water or fat soluble? What are the clinical consequences of either? Will a one and one-half inch needle deliver a medication into the muscle or into the fatty tissue? Should intramuscular injection even be attempted? What are the effects of opioids on senso-

### ACUTE AND CHRONIC PAIN

Acute pain is short term, lasting form seconds to months. The source of the pain could be inflammation, tissue damage, injury, or surgery, and usually resolves when the underlying cause or source has resolved. This type of pain can interfere with recovery as pain often signals danger, and therefore patients may be reluctant to participate in even the most basic care. In the presence of chronic pain, acute pain can be difficult to assess and manage properly.

Chronic pain makes living a normal life nearly impossible, because sometimes it lasts a lifetime. Chronic pain may be due to nerve damage, cancer, arthritis, or other reason. It affects many people, especially the obese person, and is a major cause of disability. Chronic pain may be constant or intermittent and holds physical, psychological, social, and spiritual consequences. Dealing with chronic pain can lead to depression and often leads to emotional pain. Hospitalized patients who experience acute pain superimposed onto chronic pain can pose numerous issues, and hospitalized patients who experience emotional pain are even more challenging. It is imperative for clinicians to recognize the need for respect, acceptance, and support in dealing with the complexities of the obese patient. Preoperative assessment is necessary to determine the level of chronic pain prior to surgery. A comprehensive understanding of pharmaceutical and non-pharmaceutical options for pain management is important, and strategies to minimize emotional pain should be included in the plan of care.

rium or already compromised pulmonary function? What role does long-term chronic pain have on the surgical patient's interpretation of acute pain? How is this assessed preoperatively (See: Acute or Chronic Pain)? Finally, is postoperative nausea among morbidly obese patients due to the type of surgery performed or a side effect of the medication? These largely unanswered questions further complicate pain management among the obese patient. In many cases, pain can lead to behaviors that

appear to be health-defeating activities.

### UNDERSTANDING PAIN

Overcoming the myths and misinformation that abound regarding pain assessment and treatment is one of the greatest challenges to pain management.[7] Pain is a completely subjective experience. A widely used definition is that pain is whatever the experiencing person says it is and exists whenever he or she says it does.[6] The self-report of pain by a patient should be consid-

**MANAGING CHRONIC PAIN**

1. **Accept the pain: Learn everything you can about pain and how it works, recognize that there may be no cure for the pain and you may need to mange the pain throughout your life.**
2. **Get involved: Take an active role in your situation, become a partner is your care.**
3. **Set priorities: Recognize the value of your life and those areas that give you pleasure, create a plan to help you enjoy those important activities in life.**
4. **Set realistic goals: Set goals, but keep in mind that they should be small and progress incrementally.**
5. **Know your basic rights: Demand to be treated with respect, understand what you are able and unable to accomplish, avoid feeling guilty**
6. **Recognize emotions: The physical and emotional self are really one entity, and therefore emotional pain can contribute to physical pain.**
7. **Learn to relax: pain can be aggravated by stress, learn stress triggers, and those that promote relaxation**
8. **Exercise: Unused muscles can lead to unnecessary pain; consider a modest level of physician approved activity.**
9. **See the total picture: Do not allow pain to become the center of your life—learn to set priorities, reach goals, assert basic rights, manage feelings, relax and gain control of your body.**
10. **Reach out: Many people experience chronic pain, and we learn form one another, once pain is managed reach out to others to give and receive support.**

**Adapted from: Managing Chronic Pain: Ten steps from Patient to Person. Available at: www.theacpa.org.**

ered sufficient evidence to establish the presence of pain. Acceptance of pain as a subjective experience is difficult for many healthcare professions. Often old paradigms continue to pose barriers to adequate pain control. Inadequate documentation tools fail to communicate pain and pain ratings. A pharmacist and pain specialist are essential in determining the most appropriate drug based on absorption mechanisms and rates, which can be complicated by the patient's adiposity. The unique needs of the obese patient are especially important in making a drug selection and interpreting the consequences of the chosen medication.

## *CONSIDERING ROUTES*

In many settings, use of the intramuscular route is widespread, despite the fact that research suggests that the intravenous or intraspinal (intrathecal) route for analgesics is usually safer and more effective.[8] In the bariatric patient, it may be impossible to deliver an intramuscular (IM) injection because of the presence of a thick layer of fatty tissue. The IM route may not provide predictable levels of drugs and therefore is not recommended.[9] Intravenous (IV) infusion can sometimes be challenging simply because IV access itself can be difficult. Veins may be located deep within fatty tissue, making visualization trickier. A peripherally inserted central catheter (PICC) might be considered if IV access becomes problematic. For example, PICC is indicated to secure vascular access when peripheral venous access is limited or impossible or when IV access in necessary for days to weeks.

Intrathecal continuous infusion had been useful among bariatric patients for short-term pain management. Care should be taken if the infusion catheter exits through a deep skin fold. The intertriginous regions must be clean and dry. If signs of sign breakdown occur, the skin expert, whether a WOCN, PT/OT, physician, or other consultant, must be summoned to make recommendations as to prevention of skin injury.

The non-narcotic implantable devices are garnering attention in that they provide sufficient levels of pain control without the dangers of systemic narcotic intervention. ON-Q PainBuster (I-Flow Corporation, Lake Forest, California) is one such device that is designed to improve the recovery period by helping patients get back to normal after surgery by reducing or eliminating the need for narcotics, which is today's standard of care for pain relief. The device consists of a small balloon pump that holds a local anesthetic and a tiny, specially designed catheter that continuously delivers the anesthetic directly into the surgical site. The device is portable and can be attached to the patient's gown or placed in a carrying pouch. The infusion is designed to last 2 to 5 days, and when the infusion is complete, the catheter is removed and the pump is discarded. Currently, over 40 studies are being conducted related to non-narcotic implantable devices, and the target surgeries to date are cesarean section, hysterectomies, knee replacements, mastectomies, cardiothoracic/vascular surgeries, foot/ankle surgeries, and cosmetic procedures. Clinicians experienced in the challenges of both panniculectomy and laparoscopic BWLS are interested in this strategy, recognizing the opportunity for research specific to the obese population.

## RESPIRATORY ISSUES

The resedation phenomenon is best described by Charles Callery and Judy Davidson as a delayed response to narcotic administration. This delay is largely due to unpredictable absorption and availability of the medication. Respiratory depression is a potentially life-threatening side effect among all patients but can be especially serious among morbidly obese patients. The effects of respiratory depression can be controlled through careful monitoring of sedation levels. It is especially critical to assess for sedation levels and respiratory status when starting opioids on a patient who has moderate to severe pain and has not been receiving opioids regularly. When an opioid causes the patient to be so sedated that he or she has difficulty staying awake, the dose should be decreased to prevent respiratory depression. The likelihood of respiratory depression decreases the longer the patient has been on opioids because tolerance to respiratory depression develops and information about the patient's response to opioids is known. Consider a semi-Fowler's position if respiratory depression is suspected.

## BODY POSITION AND RESPIRATORY FUNCTION

Proper positioning can be crucial in critically ill, morbidly obese patients, both to maximize lung function and to increase the likelihood of successful weaning, said Suzanne M. Burns, RN, MSN, an Associate Professor of Nursing at the University of Virginia Health Sciences Center in Charlottesville. Burns reports that in a study of 19 obese patients being weaned from mechanical ventilation, she and her colleagues found that the 45-degree upright and reverse Trendelenburg positions were associated with better respiratory mechanics than were the 90-degree upright and supine positions. Furthermore, patients typically preferred them. "Supine is probably the worst position for these large patients," commented Professor Burns, who explained that the supine position reduces pulmonary compliance and increases airway resistance. Proning morbidly obese patients is not impossible, just difficult, she added. Evidence suggests that proning can improve functional residual capacity, pulmonary compliance, and oxygenation. Hydraulic lifts, oversized wheelchairs, and other special equipment facilitate positioning of these patients, Professor Burns said. A positive attitude and determination on the part of caregivers to position these patients properly despite their size are also essential, she emphasized.

The antidote for respiratory depression is naloxone (Narcan) administered intravenously. Naloxone is a pure opioid antagonist that can reverse both analgesic effects and respiratory depression. Sufficient amounts of naloxone should be given to decrease sedation and increase respirations to an acceptable level without completely reversing analgesia. Giving too much naloxone can also precipitate hypertension and ventricular dysrhythmias. Therefore, dilute 0.4mg of naloxone in 9- to 10mL of saline and administer 0.5mL over two minutes.

## CHRONIC PAIN

Many patients who experience long-term chronic pain become depressed and anxious. Depression and anxiety can be exacerbated if it is difficult to establish a clear physical cause for the pain. Assessment of chronic pain in the acute care setting where surgery or other experiences superimpose acute pain can be difficult for patients and clinicians. These patients may begin to question their judgment, fear they will be perceived as troublesome, and worry that pain relief will be withheld because the pain is not considered real. These emotional responses may cause some healthcare providers to think that the pain is psychogenic or not of a physiologic nature. It then becomes important for clinicians who care for obese patients to understand that physiologically, the body adapts to pain after a period of time, and vital signs normalize. This return to equilibrium is necessary to prevent physical harm and undue stress on the body. It does not necessarily mean pain has been controlled adequately. Additionally, patients might exhibit a behavioral adaptation to both acute and chronic pain. They may minimize their expressions of pain for a number of reasons. A patient may wish to be seen as a good patient or may place a personal or cultural value on a stoic response to pain. The patient may become too exhausted to respond vigorously to pain. Sometimes patients use distraction techniques to move the focus away from pain, especially when intense and unrelieved.

## ASSESSMENT CHALLENGES

Each patient's situation should be reviewed separately to determine the acceptable level of sedation and to assess the potential for harm from decreased sensorium. Some patients choose to endure more discomfort if it means less sedation. If the sedation level is still unacceptable after a few days of adaptation,

### THE SUBJECTIVE EXPERIENCE

Self-reporting of pain is the single most reliable method of assessing pain intensity, and it is used whenever possible. Vitals sings and behavior are never used in place of the patient's self-report, because they are not as accurate.

another opioid can be substituted until a satisfactory one is found.

The goal in screening for pain among bariatric patients is to include questions on the clinical admission form, such as "Do you have pain now or have you experienced any pain recently?" If most patients are cognitively intact adults, the 0-to-10 pain rating scale (0=no pain, 10=worst pain) typically is used. If chronic pain is identified preoperatively, a more comprehensive pain assessment should include location, quality, onset, frequency, and intensity. These items are self-explanatory, and it is easy to ask the patient about them. Location can be assessed by asking the patient to point to the site of pain on his or her body or on a figure drawing. To assess quality, the patient may need to be given examples of descriptive terminology, such as burning, aching, dull, knife-like, or shooting.

One purpose of pain management is to ensure sufficient relief for the patient to allow for certain therapeutic activities. Determining a comfort/function goal will do this. A comfort/function goal is established by asking the patient what pain rating would allow him or her to perform specific activities. For example, the patient in this case situation may need to ambulate three times daily to prevent

> ## PAIN MANAGEMENT TASK FORCE
>
> **A** pain care committee is one mechanism for promoting an interdisciplinary approach to improving pain management throughout an institution. The committee usually consists of 7 to 10 people and includes a nurse educator, an anesthesiologist or a certified registered nurse anesthetist, a physician, a pharmacist, and several staff nurses. Staff nurses are indispensable because pain assessment and treatment are performed by nurses at the bedside. Their input will help prevent many implementation failures, such as those that may occur when revised documentation forms are first put into use. The pain care committee usually becomes a standing committee because improving pain management is an ongoing need.

skin and pulmonary complications. The patient would be asked, "What pain rating will make it easy for you to walk with the physical therapist three times daily?" He may respond that 3 on a scale of 0-10 would be sufficient. The comfort/function goal would be documented as "3/10 to ambulate with PT." When establishing comfort/function goals, keep in mind that research has suggested that pain ratings above 4 significantly interfere with activities and mood.[13] Some patients have no reluctance to accept adequate pain management, while others need to be reminded that inadequate pain control will serve as a barrier to the recovery process.

## NAUSEA

Nausea is not uncommon following surgery. Opioids are often thought to be the source of the nausea. However, other

causes of nausea, such as non-opioid medications, hypercalcemia, uncontrolled pain, copious sputum, or co-existing medical conditions may be overlooked. Carefully review signs, symptoms, and the patient's case history before targeting opioids as the cause of nausea.

## EDUCATION

Effective pain management education is essential for patients and their families. On admission, patients should be informed, both by staff and in printed information, that effective pain relief should be provided, that they should tell staff about unrelieved pain, and that staff will quickly respond. Patients and family members need to know that inadequate pain relief can interfere with important goals, such as respiratory issues and immobility concerns. An institution may develop its own

written materials and videotapes or may obtain them from
pharmaceutical companies.
Patient-teaching pamphlets for
surgery and cancer are available from AHCPR.

## CONCLUSION

In summary, the value of an
interdisciplinary team should
not be overlooked.[14] Recovery
and rehabilitation can be
affected by uncontrolled pain,
which is an opportunity where
the patient is best managed by
a team who understands the
special needs of larger
patients. The pain specialist,
pharmacist, physician, physi-
cal/occupational therapist,
bariatric CNS, and other interested professionals are important members of the team.

Research designed to investigate the meaning of pain,
pain assessment, and management for obese patients provide opportunities for interested clinicians to pursue.
Additionally, research that
seeks to more fully understand
processes related to developing, implementing, and measuring criteria-based protocols
that provide bariatric
resources in a timely and cost-
effective manner afford investi-
gational opportunities.
Together these research
opportunities serve to begin
building evidence wherein
responsible patient care choices can be made.

## REFERENCES

1. Gallagher SM. Tailoring care for obese patients. *RN* 1999;62(5):43–5.

2. Peripherally inserted central catheter (PICC) in children. Available at: www.barttersite.com/PICCchildren.htm. Access date: May 2005.

3. Ask your surgeon: On Q pain relief. Available at: www.askyoursurgeon.com/painreliefoptions.php#e. Access date: June 2005.

4. On QPain Buster. Available at: I-Flow.com

5. Davidson J, Callery C. Care of the obesity surgery patient requiring immediate level care or intensive care. *Obes Surg* 2001;11:93–7.

6. Burns SM, Egloff MB, Ryan B, et al. Effect of body position on spontaneous respiratory rate and tidal volume in patients with obe-sity, abdominal distension and ascites. *Am J Crit Care* 1994;3:102–6.

7. Naloxone. Available at: www.rxlist.com/cgi/rxlist.cgi?drug=naloxone&imageField.x=56&imageField.y=8. Access date: June 2005.

8. Managing chronic pain. American Chronic Pain Association. Available at: www.theacpa.org/pf_02.asp. Access date: June 2005.

9. Gallagher S. Pain management, obesity and critical care. Poster presentation. Las Vegas, NV: Symposium on Advanced Wound Care, 2005.

# Sensitivity

**11**

**B**ariatrics is a relatively new and general term derived from the Greek word *baros* and refers to the practice of healthcare relating to the treatment of obesity and associated conditions.[1] The American Society for Bariatric Surgery (ASBS) defines obesity more precisely as "a lifelong, progressive, life-threatening, genetically related multifactorial disease of excess fat storage with multiple comorbidities."[2] The National Association to Advance Fat Acceptance (NAAFA) does not consider a larger person obese; they contend that this term is disapproving and medicalizes a very natural state. NAAFA reminds us that some people are born tall, some short, some skinny, and ultimately, some fat. The organization explains, "We are tired of being labeled in a negative light simply for our God-given habitus."[3] Regardless, according to the NIH, obesity is simply a diagnostic category that represents a complex and multifactorial condition.[4] Medicare has just recently acknowledged obesity as an illness, thereby paving the way for special reimbursement in some cases. Some of the healthcare problems associated with obesity can include diabetes, hypertension, soft tissue infection, some cancers, and impaired circulation, each of which impairs a person's health. These comorbidities seem to now affect some of the morbidly obese population disproportionately and at a younger age.[5]

In one sense, the cause of obesity is straightforward, which is the state of expending less energy than the amount consumed. But in another sense, obesity is intangible, involving the complex individual regulation of body weight and, specifically, body fat.[6] This individual regulation is the unknown factor in the weight management enigma.[7]

Widespread disparities exist in the statistics pertaining to weight and weight issues; these disparities are caused by the differences in region, gender, and race of the reported populations being studied. Regardless, most agree that 67 percent of Americans are overweight,[10] and 35 percent are considered obese.[8,9] Studies suggest a substantial increase in obesity among all groups, regardless of age, ethnicity, race, and socioeconomic background.[10] For example, in the

mid-20th century, only a quarter of Americans were overweight; today not only are over two-thirds of American adults overweight, but 25 percent of adolescents are considered overweight as well.

Obese people, their friends, and their family members are likely to feel economic, physical, and emotional effects in all areas of their lives. Americans spend close to $33 billion annually in attempts to control or lose weight, while $117 billion is spent on obesity-related healthcare. Despite efforts at weight loss, Americans continue to gain weight, with obesity reaching pandemic proportions. An interviewee in the Public Broadcasting Service (PBS) *Frontline: Fat* explains, "...I've tried Weight Watchers, all kinds of magazine diets, phen-fen...I have even had my jaw wired." Each weight loss experience ended with a regain of the lost weight plus more, creating bounding feelings of helplessness and hopelessness.[11]

The preoccupation with weight control and the human body is pervasive, and as some now argue, for good reason.

Obesity is a factor in 5 of the 10 leading causes of death, and while it was once considered the second most common cause of early and

preventable death in the United States, today it is the top preventable killer.[12] In addition to the physiologic costs, some authors argue that obesity is associated with emotional conditions, such as situational depression, altered self esteem, and social isolation.[13] However, other experts argue that it is society's response to the obese person that leads to these emotional conditions, and that society's response includes widespread prejudice and discrimination.[14]

## PREJUDICE AND DISCRIMINATION

The issues of weight and health are extremely complex, with medical research many times raising more questions than providing answers. Because of the pressure to be thin, many obese Americans have a history of gaining and losing weight, which is the phenomenon described as "weight cycling." Certainly there are health risks inherent in being overweight; however, emotional and physical risks are extremely high in weight cycling. Although research suggests that it may be healthier to maintain a stable weight than to yo-yo diet, most overweight or obese people have a history of the repeated losing and regaining of weight, a behavior perpetuated by the continued social pressure to lose weight, thus avoiding widespread social prejudice and discrimination.

Although related, the terms *prejudice* and *discrimination* hold very different meanings. Prejudice is described as a prejudgment, and arguably most people carry some form of prejudgment toward a particular category of individuals or group. On the other hand, discrimination refers to behavior based on this prejudgment. Overweight Americans experience both.

Extensive investigation into biases regarding obesity in general and the obese person specifically suggests that this type of prejudice and discrimination crosses employment, education, and other important life-sustaining activities.[15] Research suggests that prejudice toward obese people develops at a very young age. For example, children as young as age six describe silhouettes of obese children as lazy, stupid, and ugly. According to the same study, prejudice toward the obese child is observed regardless of race or socioeconomic status.[16] Children are not the only ones who hold a prejudice directed toward the overweight person; these attitudes are as evident in adulthood. One study found that

**WEBSOURCES**

- **American Society for Bariatic Surgeons—www.asbs.org. Professional organization for surgeons and allied health professionals interested in improving care for the obese patient having BWLS.**

- **National Association for the Advancement of Fat Acceptance— www.naafa.org. Valuable site for size and weight acceptance activists, and sponsors of the "Say No to Diet Day."**

- **Council for Size and Weight Discrimination—www.cswd.org. Important consumer-driven resource for larger Americans; size and weight advocates.**

- **Obesity Help—www.obesityhelp.com. Resource for consumers and healthcare providers offering education and "chat" opportunities.**

- **The Rudd Insititute—www.yale.edu/rudd. The Rudd Institute uses the moniker "See the person, not the pounds" as it provides support and resources for sensitivity, understanding, and education pertaining to weight and weight issues.**

although college students rate their obese peers as warm and friendly, they also rate them as unhappy, lacking in self confidence, self indulgent, and undisciplined compared to their nonobese peers.[17] In another study, obese students were described as less active, less intelligent, less hardworking, less attractive, less popular, less successful, less athletic, and less appropriately sextyped than the nonobese.[18]

Healthcare clinicians are also often biased against the larger patient.[19] In using the Bray Attitudes Toward Obesity Survey (BATOS) to measure attitudes of dietitians toward obese patients, bias was even observed among obese persons themselves.[20] Health professionals are far from immune to these culturally driven views. In one study wherein mental health professionals were asked to evaluate identical case histories with corresponding photographs of either normal weight or obese women, the obese women were rated significantly higher on agitation-impaired judgment, inadequate hygiene, inappropriate behavior, intolerance of change, stereotyped behavior, suspicion, and total psychological dysfunction.[21] Another study incorporated use of the "fat suit," which was used to change the appearance of patients. A videotaped session featured the same patient with and without the fat suit. Medical students reported that the patient masquerading as the obese person was more defensive, nervous, insincere, seductive, depressed, emotional, cold, and unlikable than when appearing as nonobese.[22] Despite the growing body of medical research that suggests otherwise, many health professionals continue to believe that obesity is a self-inflicted condition that results from a lack of will power.[23]

This discrimination leads to profound economic consequences. Research has shown a correlation between obesity and lower socioeconomic status, especially among women.[24] It has been assumed that the obesity is caused by low socioeconomic status, but several studies present evidence that the reverse is true—that low socioeconomic status is caused by obesity.[25] For example, in a study that followed overweight and normal weight adolescents for seven years, as the adolescents reached maturity, researchers found that the overweight women were less educated, less likely to marry, and had

lower household incomes and higher rates of household poverty than women who were of healthy weight. These differences were independent of baseline aptitude test scores and initial socioeconomic status. In another study that compared subjects' current incomes with those of their parents at the time the subjects were eight years old, the obese men and women were more likely to have lower incomes than their parents than the non-obese men and women. Again, this suggests that obesity causes poverty and not vice versa.[26]

The argument is made by some that obese people are not given the same opportunities as the nonobese. The obese are less likely than the nonobese to be accepted into colleges and universities. The obese applied at the same rate as the nonobese and the applicants did not differ in academic performance, scholastic aptitude test scores, IQ scores, class rank, number of days absent, visits to the school nurse, motivation to attend college, parental income, or involvement in extracurricular activities. The obese were simply denied admission more often than the nonobese.

The same patterns hold true when the obese enter the work force. For example,

when job applications were accompanied by either a photograph or written description of the candidate, written descriptions of the obese applicants include more negative stereotyping. Similarly, when judged on their desirability as employees, obese persons are viewed as less competent, disorganized, indecisive, inactive, less likely to take initiative, less likely to persevere, and more likely to possess poor self discipline than candidates who were underweight or of average weight. Thus, employment discrimination against the obese is many times based on these types of prejudgments and overlooks actual ability.

Historically, obesity has been perceived as a problem of self discipline.[27] However, recent discoveries suggest that this may in fact be far from the truth. For example, consider the Pima Indian groups in the southwestern US. They are thought to possess what James Neel refers to as the "thrifty gene." Over centuries of evolution, this group survived in part by very efficiently metabolizing their calories, providing for long periods of famine. Today, the genetically homogenous group living south of the US/Mexican border maintains an average of 22 hours of intense activity each week. Most members of this community eat the indigenous diet, and have no problem with obesity; however, those living north of the border in the US have adopted the western diet, which is high in fat, high in calories, and high in carbohydrates. To compound the problem, this group in general has adopted the sedentary lifestyle of many Americans. The Pima Indian people are experiencing profound levels of obesity, diabetes, hypertension, and all the complications inherent in morbid obesity.[28] There is no debate about the statement that weight gain occurs when intake (food intake) exceeds output (activity); the real mystery behind balancing body weight depends on a number of other factors. Genetics, gender, physiology, biochemistry, neuroscience, as well as cultural, environmental, and psychosocial factors influence weight and its regulation.[29] Healthcare clinicians best serve their patients when they recognize obesity as a multifactorial chronic condition.

Obese Americans neither chose to be overweight nor chose to experience the widespread prejudices and discrimination that is prevalent in American society today.[30] Failure to provide appropriate intervention is often based on the premise that inadequate policies and procedures are

## THE VOICE OF THE PATIENT

As a very outgoing slim child, I was ill prepared for my developing adolescent body. As I entered my teens, my weight just got away from me. At only 5'2" tall and 225 pounds, I could no longer comfortably sit at my desk at school, wear ready-made clothes, ride in my brother's compact car, or work behind the counter at the grill where I was employed 12 hours a week. For several years I became very isolated and withdrawn, and I no longer socialized with friends or family members outside of my home. I failed to fit in at every turn, and my weight soared to 400 pounds by the time I was 17 years old.

My parents helped me in many ways. After years of struggle, I now weigh 185 pounds. I know I am still very heavy, but I fit in. I went to nursing school, and I work in the newborn nursery. I know I look very maternal and, therefore, in my mind, I feel that the new parents accept me more readily...and so do my colleagues.

When I learned the hospital was developing a task force to examine needs of very large patients, I welcomed the opportunity to join the team. It has been 12 months now and work on the team has been slow because of the complexities of the institution, but also because of the complexities of the patients' needs. I believe I am a very valuable member of the team in that I keep the team focused on the actual needs of larger patients. I serve as a constant reminder to maintain a size-appropriate and, therefore sensitive environment for a vulnerable population. For example, we ordered really beautiful armchairs for the bariatric patient suites that were built to accommodate a 500-pound patient or visitor; however, because of the width of the chair, when I sat my 185-pound body into it, the arms pressed uncomfortably into my hips. The goal of the team is to better meet the emotional and physical needs of the bariatric patient, and without the input of a larger person it makes it more difficult to accomplish this goal.

justified by blaming the patient for his or her condition. A primary role of the healthcare clinicians in caring for this vulnerable population is to guarantee a safe haven from the obesity-related prejudice and discrimination, which often stems from misunderstandings of the nature and cause of obesity.

In addition, one study that examined caregiver attitudes toward the BWLS patient suc-

cessfully linked inadequate tools for providing care with negative attitudes toward the patient. Rather than simply exploring verbal prejudice, the focus of this study examined failure to provide reasonable accommodation in the form of medical equipment, comfortable surroundings, properly fitting attire, etc. This particular study suggested that bias exists toward the morbidly obese patient despite the

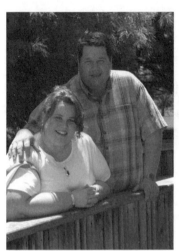

**Special training in the care of the obese patient is essential. Discussions on the use of oversized equipment, sensitivity, mobility techniques, pathophysiology, and pain management will better prepare clinicians to understand the complex needs of the patient.**

degree of overweight. The same study also found that most hospital departments treated patients well, except for those with equipment that was insufficiently sized to safely meet the patient's needs.[31]

The concern of prejudice and discrimination is that these emotions pose barriers to healthcare regardless of the practice setting or professional discipline. The overwhelming misunderstanding of obesity is likely to interfere with preplanning efforts, access to services, and resource allocation. Although this misunderstanding is not universal, it is

pervasive enough to pose obstacles, and clinicians interested in making changes need to acknowledge this barrier. It is interesting that the department most ill prepared to handle patients was thought to hold the greatest bias. Perhaps introduction of appropriate preplanning efforts can play a role in improving the level of compassion, sensitivity, and understanding in caring for the larger, heavier, and more complex patient.

## IMPLICATIONS IN THE HEALTHCARE SETTING

Despite education, clinical skills, and motivation, challenges to delivering safe, effective, patient-centered care for the obese exist. Clinicians across the country and across practice settings recognize that threats to compassion, sensitivity, and understanding will continue to pose barriers until caregiver-safe strategies for care are available. Even the most compassionate caregiver may be reluctant to provide adequate care because of the threat of caregiver injury. This realistic fear of injury, along with the failure to provide satisfactory care to a complex patient, further perpetuates discrimination toward the obese patient.

To properly recognize the value of removing these barri-

ers toward care and implementing preplanning for the heavier, more complex patient, we must first discuss the meaning and significance of obesity in America. A considerable amount of tension arises from issues of weight, whether the discussion concerns anorexia, bulimia, or obesity. And despite the fact that these eating disorders are really a preoccupation with food, which is a different side of the same coin, obesity carries the most significant social stigma. Healthcare clinicians, as members of society at large, are likely to carry the same bias toward obesity as the general population. Instead of investigating ways to provide the most comprehensive care possible, clinicians face colleagues who ask why patients allow themselves to become so heavy, or why weight loss is not the primary goal in care. A well-meaning clinician suggesting weight loss to an obese person without an in depth knowledge of the many tools available is like asking a carpenter to repair a cabinet with a single hammer. The etiologies of obesity are complex and multifactorial, and management options should reflect this. Such misunderstandings suggest that as a culture, we need to be more aware of the moral dimensions of weight issues and recognize how they not only influence the physical and emotional being, but most importantly how they influence the direct physical care of the obese patient.

Policies and procedures are designed to ensure a standardized method of delivering care based on specific criteria. Although preplanning for equipment is an essential first step, it simply is not sufficient to adequately prevent the costly, predictable complications that occur in caring for obese patients. A comprehensive and interdisciplinary patient care approach may be necessary to provide safe patient care, and prevent caregiver injury in a timely, cost-effective manner. The approach should include: 1) a bariatric task force, 2) criteria-based protocol, 3) competencies and skills set, and 4) outcome measurement efforts.

The **bariatric task force** is an interdisciplinary quality improvement effort designed to address ongoing issues and ideas.[32] The value of an interdisciplinary approach, which includes a patient representative, cannot be overlooked (See: The Voice of the Patient). Pharmacists, physical/occupational and respiratory therapists, physicians, clinical nurse specialists, counselors, social workers, risk managers, and others can

---

**MEASUREMENT TOOLS**

**IMPLICIT ASSOCIATION TEST (IAT) is a timed measure of automatic association of a target construct with particular attributes. Unlike self-report questionnaires, the IAT is designed to assess associations that exist beyond conscious evaluation, providing a measurement of automatic biases of which people are unaware or unwilling to report. implicit.harvard.edu/implicit/demo**

**BRAY ATTITUDE TOWARD OBESITY SURVEY (BATOS) is a 40-item, Likert, easily scored, self-assessment tool designed to measure attitudes toward obesity among all areas of specialty or discipline. See the BATOS used in: Maiman LA, Wang VL, Becker MH, et al. Attitudes toward obesity and the obese among professionals. *J Am Diet Assoc* 1979;74:331–6.**

---

be essential in planning care. Each member of the team brings a unique and important perspective.[33] Operating as a cohesive unit, the entire healthcare team must be diligent in caring for the morbidly obese patient.

All healthcare facilities should have a plan in place for the special needs of the morbidly obese patient. A **criteria-based protocol** is simply preplanning based on specifically designated criterion.[34] The patient's weight, body mass index (BMI), body width, and clinical condition serve as such criteria. A first step is to determine the weight limit of equipment the patient is likely to need. This might include operating room tables, wheelchairs, radiology equipment, wall-mounted toilets, and furniture in the room and lobby. Healthcare facilities should ask members

of the task force to look around their work areas to locate equipment the patient will utilize. The actual weight of the patient and the weight limit of the equipment is particularly useful, because if the weight limit of equipment is exceeded, then breakage, failure to properly function, or patient/caregiver injury can occur. Body width is described as the patient's body at his or her widest point, which can be at the patient's hips, shoulders, or across the belly when sidelying.

Understanding potential complications and corresponding interventions is a large part of caregivers possessing the **competency/skills set** necessary to prevent risks to patient, visitors, and caregivers. Communication and timing is critical to prevent these hazards. Although sometimes difficult to arrange, a face-to-face inter-disciplinary conference, which is planned within 24 hours of admission, may prevent costly intervention later.[35] Consider including the patient's spouse or significant other, as this person may offer insight into the patient's individual emotional, spiritual, or physical needs. Careful documentation of meetings, individual goals, and corresponding intervention may protect the institution from legal action. This level of accountability also more fully outlines each clinician's responsibilities and, when the timing is right, also smoothes the patient transition from one practice setting to another.

Special training in the care of the obese patient is essential. Discussions on the use of oversized equipment, sensitivity, mobility techniques, pathophysiology, and pain management will better prepare clinicians to understand the complex needs of the patient.[36]

Finally, **outcome measurement efforts** are especially helpful in determining the actual impact that the comprehensive program has on cost, clinical outcomes, and satisfaction outcomes. Consider evaluating attitudes toward obesity before and after introduction of such

preplanning activities (See: Measurement Tools).

## CONCLUSION

Modern culture idealizes thin and disparages obesity.[40] It is possible that in healthcare settings, this dynamic may be more intense simply because of the challenges in lifting, repositioning, turning, or difficulty in the general care of the obese patient.

Numerous resources are available to clinicians across practice settings, and use of resources in a timely and appropriate manner are thought to improve measurable therapeutic, satisfaction, and cost outcomes, including attitudes. The obese patient presents many care challenges, and it is in the interest of all stakeholders, including insurance carriers, healthcare organizations, clinicians, patients, and their families to consider preplanning opportunities. It is also in the spirit of comprehensive clinical care to understand that the failure to preplan for this care affects attitudes toward this vulnerable population.

## REFERENCES

1.  Gallagher S. Bariatrics: Considering mobility, patient safety, and caregiver injury. In: Charney W, Hudson A (eds). *Back Injury Among Healthcare*. CRC Press 2004.
2.  American Society for Bariatric Surgery. Available at: www.asbs.org. Access date: June 2004.
3.  National Association for the Advancement of Fat Acceptance. Available at: www.naafa.org. Access date: August 2004.
4.  Kuczmarski RJ, Fiegel KM, Campbell SM, Johnson CL. Increasing prevalence of overweight among US adults. The National Health and Nutrition Examination surveys, 1960 to 1991. *J Am Med Assoc* 1994;272:205–11.
5.  Kral JG, Strauss RJ, Wise L. Perioperative risk management in obese patients. In: Deitl M. *Surgery for the Morbidly Obese Patient*. North York (Canada): FD Communications, 2000.
6.  Gallagher S, Arzouman J, Lacovara J, et al. Criteria-based protocols and the obese patient: Planning care for a high-risk population. *Ostomy Wound Manage* 2004;50:32–42.
7.  Gallagher S. Taking the weight off with bariatric surgery. *Nursing* 2004;34:58–64.
8.  Gallagher S. Meeting the needs of the obese patient. *AJN* 1996;96:1s–12s.
9.  Rippe JM. The obesity epidemic: challenges and opportunities. *J AM Diet Assoc* 1998.98(suppl 2):S5.
10. Lanz P, House J, Lepowski J et al. Socioeconomic factors, health behavior and mortality. *JAMA* 1998;279:1703–8.
11. (ed). *Frontline: Fat PBS Home Video*. Seattle: Public Broadcasting Service, 1998.
12. Fox HR. Discrimination: Alive and well in the United States. *Obes Surg* 1995;5:352.
13. Charles S. Psychological evaluation of morbidly obese patients. *Gastro Clinics of North Am* 1987;16:415–32.
14. (ed). *Frontline Fat PBS Home Video*. Seattle: Public Broadcasting Service;1998.
15. Faulcbaum L, Choban P. Surgical implications of obesity. *Annu Rev Med* 1998;49:215–34.
16. Staffieri JR. A study of social stereotype of body image in children. *JPers Soc Psychol* 1967;7:101–4.
17. Tiggemann M, Rothblum ED. Gender differences in social consequences of perceived overweight. *Sex Roles* 1988;18:75–86.
18. Harris MB, Harris RJ, Bochner S. Fat, four-eyed and female:

Stereotypes of obesity, glasses and gender. *J Applied Social Psychol* 1982;12:503–16.

19. Thone RR. *Fat: A Fate Worse Than Death*. New York: Harrington Park Press, 1997.

20. Maiman LA, Wang VL, Becker MH, et al. Attitudes toward obesity and the obese among professionals. *J Am Diet Assoc* 1979;74:331–6.

21. Young LM, Powell B. The effects of obesity on clinical judgments of mental health professionals. *J Health Soc Behav* 1985;26:233–46.

22. Breytspraak LM, McGee J, Conger JC, et al. Sensitizing medical students to impression formation processes in the patient interview. *J Med Educ* 1977;52:47–54.

23. Falkner NH, French SA, Jeffrey RW, et al. Mistreatment due to weight: Prevalence and sources of perceived mistreatment in women and men. *Obes Res* 1999;7:572–6.

24. Gortmaker SL, Must A, Perrin JM. Social and economic consequences of overweight in adolescence and young adulthood. *NEJM* 1993; 329:1008–19.

25. Pagan JA, Davila A. Obesity, occupational attainment, and earnings. *Soc Sci Quar* 1997;78:756–70.

26. Gortmaker SL, Must A, Perrin JM. Social and economic consequences of overweight in adolescence and young adulthood. *NEJM* 1993;329;1008–19.

27. Gallagher S. A Tragic Case of Childhood Obesity. Michigan:UMC Press, 2000.

28. NIDDK. *The Pima Indians: Pathfinders for health.* Available at: www.niddk.nih.gov/health/diabetes/pima/pathfind/pathfind.htm. Access date: August 2004.

29. Gustafson NJ. *Managing Obesity and Eating Disorders*. Western Schools Press;1997:13–19.

30. Gustafson NJ. *Managing Obesity and Eating Disorders*. Western Schools Press;1997:2.

31. Kaminsky J, Gadaleta D. A study of discrimination within the medical community as viewed by obese patients. *Obes Surg* 2002:12:14–18.

32. Gallagher S, Langlois C, Spacht D, et al. Preplanning for skin and wound care among obese patients. *Adv Skin Wound Care* 2004.

33. Gallagher S. Bariatrics: Considering mobility, patient safety, and caregiver injury. In:

Charney W., Hudson A (eds). *Back Injury Among Healthcare Workers.* Baton Rouge, LA: Lewis Publishers, 2004.

34. Gallagher S. Restructuring the therapeutic environment to promote care and safety for the obese patient. *JWOCN* 1999. 26:292–7.

35. DeRuiter HP, Meitteunen E, Sauder K. Improving safety for caregivers through collaborative practice. *Jour Healthcare Safety Compliance Infec Contr* 2001;5:61–4.

36. Gallagher S (ed). Basic nursing competencies in caring for the obese patient. Proceedings of the Symposium Advanced Wound Care; 2003 Apr 10–14;Las Vegas, NV.

37. Flegal KM, Carroll MD, Ogden CL, Johnson CL. Prevalence and trends in obesity among US adults 1990–2000. *J Am Med Assoc* 2002;288:1723–7.

## ADDITIONAL READING

1. Crandall CS, Schiffhaur KL. Anti-fat prejudice: Beliefs, values, and American culture. *Obes Res* 1998;6:458–60.

2. Fontaine KR, Bartlet SJ. Access and use of medical care among obese persons. *Obes Res* 2000;8:403–6.

3. Miller CT, Downey KT. A meta-analysis of heavyweight people and self-esteem. *Personality and Social Psychology Review* 1999;3:68–84.

4. Miller CT, Myers AM. Compensating for prejudice: How heavyweight people and others control outcomes despite prejudice. In: *Prejudice: The Target's Perspective*. 1998;191–218.

5. Solovay S. *Tipping the scales of injustice: Fighting weight based discrimination.* Amherst (NY): Prometheus Books;2000.

6. Wadden TA, Anderson DA, Foster GD, et al. Obese women's perceptions of their physicians' weight management attitudes and practices. *Archives of Fam Med* 2000;9:854–60.

# Bariatric Resources Across the Continuum

Over two-thirds of Americans are overweight, and 10 to 25 percent are obese.[1] Heavier patients are more complex and time consuming to care for, staffing seldom accommodates this difference, and reimbursement does not accommodate at all. Clinicians in the settings of home, hospital, outpatient, long-term care, and acute rehabilitation have concerns about caring for very large patients. Regardless of the practice setting, preplanning becomes essential.[2] Therefore, hospitals across the country are initiating bariatric task forces in hopes of designing processes to control or prevent some of the costly complications associated with caring for the obese patient.[3] The challenge to these groups has been the limited availability of resources on which to build. This chapter presents practical solutions to some of the costly and preventable complications of care across the continuum of care. Adequate nutritional support, IV access, skin and wound considerations, appropriate-sized equipment, airway and ventilatory management, resuscitation and diagnostic testing, pain control, social and emotional concerns, and the prevention of complications all present special and unique difficulties. These difficulties will require specific and unique approaches to assessment and data collection, development of a care plan and consistent implementation of that plan. This chapter includes the story of a composite patient who is followed from the time the 911 call is placed until the he is discharged from the home care service. Practical resources, such as longer gloves, wider commodes, specialized tracheostomy tubes, and heavy duty furniture, are provided. Real life challenges such as physical transfers, intubation, surgery, skilled nursing placement, and home care, are presented.

## BARRIERS TO CARE

In American culture, making generalizations about individuals or groups is not uncommon.[4] Many people believe that obesity occurs because of a lack of discipline or poor self control. As a result, larger Americans are frequently the object of prejudice and discrimination.[5] They may be viewed as lazy and unlikable by their leaner counterparts and very often by themselves as well. Both the larger patients and their fami-

> ### CONSIDERING COLOSTOMY CARE
>
> **J**oe has a temporary loop colostomy for 12 weeks. He was in critical care for a considerable amount of time, with significant deconditioning. He only cared for the colostomy for three weeks independently before surgical closure. Colostomy care among obese patients is of particular concern. The colostomy may be recessed or retracted, may be located within a skin fold, or is an area not visible to the patient. Gates talks about the specific issues that arise when caring for the obese patient with a colostomy. She reminds readers that preoperatively, a CWOCN consultation is imperative in determining the ideal site for the stoma, and postoperative care must actively address pain management, immobility, skin injury, respiratory issues, embolic threats, and caregiver injury. For more on specific colostomy care techniques among obese patients, please see: Gallagher S, Gates J. Challenges of ostomy care and obesity. *Ostomy Wound Manage* 2004;50:38–49.

lies need acceptance, support, and encouragement.

Hospitalized patients complain of lack of privacy and loss of control. Those who are independent at home often become dependent because of unfamiliar surroundings. Many obese patients are embarrassed because of their size and personal appearance.[6] Because of problems related to immobility, dependence, and embarrassment, these needs may be more intense once the patient is hospitalized.[7] Like all patients, the obese patient brings fears, expectations, and emotional needs to the healthcare experience.[8]

## CASE STUDY

Joe is a 54-year-old high school teacher. His body mass index (BMI) is 52, and he weighs 425 pounds. He is considered to be in good health and is independent in his activities of daily living. He is popular with his students and their parents. While at home in his upstairs bedroom, he developed severe abdominal pain. His cordless telephone was not in its cradle. As he descended the stairs, he tripped and fell, breaking his left ankle.

Paramedics had difficulty with Joe's care from the time they arrived at his home. Clinicians across the continuum were challenged by the complex nature of Joe's care.

## EMERGENCY MEDICAL SERVICES (EMS)

One paramedic confided that the real issue in transporting a very large, critically ill patient is the amount of time needed to make the transport. EMS personnel do not want to expend this degree of resources with one patient, because without appropriate equipment and preplanning, these services can become very costly to the paramedic company. In privately run services, dispatchers learn the names and addresses of the very heavy patients and might make every effort to avoid providing service. This is the unspoken but very real concern. Care may be delayed simply because EMS has become overwhelmed with the unreimbursed costs in managing a complex patient. In Joe's case, the challenge to paramedics was not only weight limits on transport equipment, but Joe's intense abdominal and left ankle pain. It becomes more difficult to transport patients who cannot cooperate because of pain. Paramedics equipped with standard-sized equipment are not able to obtain accurate blood pressure readings, and starting an IV is difficult; however, the most significant challenge is lifting a patient like Joe into the transport van. Theoretically, Joe could be placed directly onto the ambulance floor, but this causes skin trauma. When placed directly on the floor, the patient is not secured, and in the unlikely event of a traffic collision, Joe and the paramedic personnel are at risk for serious injury. Even if Joe was secured to a standard sized gurney, problems could occur. Often the upper body weight can be so great that the head of the gurney cannot be elevated. In the presence of obstructive sleep apnea or obesity hypoventilation syndrome, failure to raise the head of the gurney could result in respiratory distress or failure, compounding an already dangerous situation.

## EMERGENCY DEPARTMENT

Emergency department nurses report difficulty in assessment, diagnostic testing, and clinical intervention. Joe was particularly challenging in that in addition to severe abdominal pain, he was experiencing lower leg pain, which also impaired his mobility. Some hospital staff members report obese patients are placed directly on a mattress on the floor. This is inappropriate for the bariatric patient who may need to be placed in a semi-Fowler's position to breathe. Once on the floor, transferring the patient to a gurney is impossible, not to mention ergonomically challenging. Appropriately sized gurneys or frames with support surfaces must be available.

Pain relief was a consideration early in the emergency department experience for Joe. But excess body fat can alter drug absorption, depending on the medication. For example, diazepam and carbamazepine are highly soluble in fat and are, therefore, absorbed mostly in adipose tissue. Dosage of these drugs must be calculated using the patient's actual body weight. Drugs that are absorbed mainly into lean tissue, such as acetaminophen, should be calculated using the patient's ideal body weight.[9] Trying to remember what drugs fall into what categories is almost impossible. A clinical pharmacist can be an important resource to ensure that the drug dose is accurate.

Standard 1 to 1 1/2-inch needles may not be able to penetrate past the adipose tissue in a patient with especially thick hips. In this case, a longer needle is needed to deliver an intramuscular dosage of the intended medication, or the clinicians should consider a drug that uses another route.

A thick layer of adipose tissue interferes with visualization and location of veins, which makes it technically more difficult to identify common landmarks; therefore, inserting an IV catheter can be difficult. Some nurses report difficulty gauging depth. If it requires more than two attempts, consider using a peripherally inserted central catheter (PICC) or a midline catheter instead of a standard peripheral catheter. Placement of lines, in a non-emergency situation, can be best achieved using portable bedside ultrasound guidance.[10] Both types of catheters can stay in place for weeks or months at a time, thereby eliminating the need to repeatedly stick the patient.[10]

Blood pressure cuffs must be the proper size to fit the patients correctly. Cuffs that are too small and taped to keep them on the arm will display higher readings.[11] It is not only important to have the oversized blood pressure cuff, but staff needs to know where to locate it. Imagine Joe's embarrassment when he hears, "Where is that really big blood pressure cuff? You remember—we used it on the huge blonde lady last week." Equipment must be readily and discreetly accessible.

## SURGERY

Joe presented with two surgical needs: repair of his left ankle fracture and exploratory laparotomy for severe abdominal pain. Depending on the patient's weight and distribution, a standard operating room (OR) table may not accommodate the patient properly. Some hospitals reportedly have created an extension that is

placed on the table; however, this could interfere with the complex functions of the table. Others report that an oversized bed is used. Although this is likely to accommodate size and weight, it too precludes use of the complex functions of a specially designed OR table. Care needs to be taken to prevent pressure-related injury from straps, supports, or simply the surgeon's body resting against any tissue that extends from the table. Prevention or support table pads must be considered. A lateral transfer device may help prevent caregiver injury and reduce shearing injury that develops from moving a heavy patient from one surface to another. In fact, the risk for caregiver injury is so great with lateral transfers that some hospitals have made the decision to move the patient from the OR table directly to frame/bed that will be used for the rest of the hospitalization. If the procedure has lasted over two hours or if any discoloration of intact skin exists over the buttocks area, at the very least, a pressure relief surface should be considered.

## INTENSIVE CARE UNIT (ICU)

Joe was admitted to the intensive care unit following exploratory laparotomy, which resulted in a temporary loop

colostomy and fixation of the left ankle fracture. In the critical care settings, initial treatment is often aimed at managing the most life-threatening conditions. Ongoing treatment can extend over a prolonged period and prove difficult for the patient to tolerate. A comprehensive plan of care designed to address the specific needs of the larger patient in the critical care setting sets the tone for the remainder of the hospitalization. As in all settings, caring for Joe must target his physical, emotional, and social needs.[12] A strong collaborative effort early on that includes the patient and family members as team members can provide the most successful outcome.

Like Joe, many large people are very healthy; however, obese patients who are hospitalized for prolonged periods of time have probably been affected by a cascade of events that occur from cardiac or pulmonary complications. Complications occur because of a reduced vital capacity and increased work of breathing. This is due to a thick chest wall coupled with impaired diaphragmatic descent because of abdominal fat and elevated intra-abdominal pressure, resulting in decreased compliance.[13] Increased cardiac output and total vascular resistance are thought to be a

**HUNDREDS OF RESOURCES FOR HEAVIER PEOPLE**

Interested in hundreds of different products and resources/websources to help you plan the care of larger, heavier patients? Learn about resources from the following categories: automotive safety, bariatric surgery, brace and supports, clothing, compression garments, home care and hospital equipment, funeral and postmortem services, furniture, gloves, websources, legal service, lift chair, magazine subscriptions, maternity, motor scooter, nutritional information, operating room, patient supplies, clinic supplies and furniture, ramps, reachers, vacation resorts, scales, and transferring devices. To access this Resource Guide contact Sizewise Rentals at: *sizewise.net/1d.html.*

result of an expanded intravascular volume. This increase in left ventricular preload and afterload ultimately results in coronary insufficiency and cardiac failure. Decreased vital capacity, tidal volume, and expiratory reserve volume with increased respiratory rate are more common in the morbidly obese patient, when compared to the non-obese.[14] Postoperatively, this may result in a slower surgical recovery and development of respiratory complications. Illness, even relatively minor, in the morbidly obese can result in major catastrophes and life-threatening situations requiring urgent medical intervention and physiological support.[15-17]

Sleep apnea is found in normal weight individuals, but is more prevalent in the obese because of excess upper body weight.[18] A diagnosis of sleep apnea is made when the patient has five or more obstructive apneic episodes per hour of sleep.[19] Sleep apnea may be obstructive, central, or mixed. Co-existing symptoms include restless sleep, snoring, and daytime somnolence.[20] Hypersomnolence is characteristic and is often associated with apneic pauses during sleep, a condition that increases with progressive weight gain.[21]

Weight control is critical to good health. However, to be successful long term, timing is important. Pressure to lose weight in the midst of a critical illness is rarely necessary. However, in the face of a life-threatening, weight-sensitive respiratory condition, such as obstructive sleep apnea (OSA) or obesity hypoventilation syndrome (OHS), weight loss during an acute illness may be necessary.[22] The basis for treatment of OHS is weight reduction. Fortunately

Joe had no symptoms of OHS or OHA; however, many patients with sleep apnea have complete remission at a critical reduced weight level. Below the critical weight they are asymptomatic; however, above this weight, apneic episodes recur.[23] The percentage of weight loss needed to achieve remission will vary from patient to patient; however, from a pulmonary perspective, most researchers agree that weight loss improves total lung capacity, functional residual capacity, and forced expired volume in many patients.[24]

An overweight patient is not necessarily adequately nourished because he or she may consume calorie-dense foods that are nutritionally inadequate. Therefore, it is essential that nutritional assessment and appropriate interventions be accomplished in the critical care area and not erroneously given low priority.

Because of the patient's body mass, nutritional needs are not easy to assess. Metabolic studies are very helpful in determining more specifically what level of nutritional support is most appropriate for the patient.[25] Choosing the right type of feeding is important. The goal for Joe in the ICU is to provide adequate nutritional needs taking care to keep the

$pCO_2$ within normal limits.[26] A dietitian is instrumental in providing assessment and a nutritional plan of care tailored to meet the needs of the obese patient. Nutritional assessment includes diet history, BMI, physical exam, medical and social history, and lab values, such as serum albumin, pre-albumin, serum transferrin, and lymphocyte count.[27]

In the presence of obesity, the patient's large, heavy abdominal wall causes substantially greater pressures in the abdomen. When enteric nutrition is used, care must be taken to ensure that the tube feeding is passing from the stomach and into the small intestines. The patient may be at significant risk for aspiration, especially in the presence of elevated intra-abdominal pressure and high gastric residuals. Feeding tubes passed through the pylorus can help to reduce this risk but can be very difficult to place in the obese patient.[28] Although use of the enteric route is preferred, sometimes this is not possible, and nutrition must be delivered parenterally.

Obese patients often present with atypical pressure ulcers. Pressure within skin folds can be sufficient to cause skin breakdown. Tubes and catheters burrow into skin folds, which can further erode the skin surface. The patient needs to be repositioned at least every two hours, as do tubes and catheters. Tubes should be placed so that the patient does not rest on them. Tube and catheter holders may be helpful in this step. Commercially available securing devices that can be opened and closed several times and remain in place will reduce the likelihood of skin necrosis.

Wound healing can be problematic in some obese patients. Blood supply to fatty tissues may be insufficient to provide an adequate amount of oxygen and nutrients, which can interfere with wound healing. A delay in wound healing can occur if the patient has a diet that lacks protein or essential vitamins and nutrients. Wound healing can also be delayed if the wound is within a skin fold, where excess moisture and bacteria can accumulate. Furthermore, excess body fat increases tension at wound edges.[30] To reduce the occurrence of abdominal wound separation, some clinicians use a surgical binder to support the area. The binder will need to be large enough to comfortably fit the patient.

During the day, there was little problem locating resources to mobilize Joe; however, at night there was insufficient staff in the eight-bed intensive care unit to adequately reposition Joe when he was unable cooperate because of pain and sedation. A lift and transfer system was used to transfer him to a chair, commode, or gurney, despite staff limitations.

## RETHINKING SPACE, EQUIPMENT, AND PHYSICAL RESOURCES

Healthcare facilities need to rethink the space required to provide quality care for larger patients because of the increasing risk to patients, their families, and members of the clinical staff. Most existing architectural designs, furnishings, and equipment accommodates to 300 pounds. But what about those patients exceeding those weight limits? Problems include insufficient door widths, inadequate space to manipulate oversized equipment, inadequate space in bathrooms, and undersized diagnostic equipment. Healthcare professionals including risk managers, ergonomists, attorneys, and employee health clinicians are looking at cost-effective ways to manage these challenges. For more on the topic see: Kramer K & Gallagher S. WOC nurses as advocates for patients who are morbidly obese: A case study promoting use of bariatric beds. *Journal of Wound, Ostomy and Continence Nursing* 2004;31:276-81. Also see Muir ML & Haney LL. Designing space for the bariatric patient. *Nursing Homes/Long Term Care Management* 2004:24 -8.

In the normal weight patient, the trachea is close to the skin surface and easily located. Tracheostomy surgery in the morbidly obese patient can be technically difficult. The term bull neck is used to describe a short, thick neck with excessive fat, which is common among obese patients. This unique anatomic configuration presents a surgical challenge. It may be necessary to create a large, deep tracheotomy incision in order to localize the trachea, which may be buried deep beneath fatty tissue.

Management problems that arise from tracheostomy surgery include care of a large, deep wound, securing the trach tube, management of drainage, protection of surrounding intact skin, and care of the tracheostomy tube.[31] The wound is vulnerable to infection because of its size, the presence of respiratory secretions, and poor vascularity of adipose tissue.

Wound cleansing with normal saline or a commercially prepared wound cleanser will reduce bacterial load within the wound. Local wound care may be complicated because of its close proximity to the airway. When selecting a wound dressing, it is important that the wound dressing does not deteriorate or dislodge, which could occlude or be aspirated into the airway.

Although the skin is a natural barrier to infection, irritation from excessive moisture from tracheal secretions can cause denuding of surrounding intact skin and lead to cellulitis, candidiasis, and discomfort to the patient. For example, consider Sara, a 380-pound patient in the critical care unit who, unlike Joe, has a tracheostomy, which was performed to relieve symptoms of OSA. The peristomal wound measures 10cm x 2cm. Daily care entails cleansing the wound with normal saline. A nonadherent, moisture-absorbing foam dressing was tucked under the tracheostomy tube holder. The extra-wide foam tie with a Velcro fastening system is especially helpful in larger patients as it extends to 25 inches in length. A 4in x 4in gauze dressing was placed over the foam dressing to absorb excessive moisture. The gauze was changed as needed when moist. The principles that directed the wound care were to reduce bacterial load by cleansing with a noncytotoxic agent, such as normal saline (NS) or a wound cleanser, cover the wound with a dressing that maintains its integrity and protects the surgical wound from external irritants, and secure the tracheotomy tube using ties that do not cause additional cutaneous injury.

Maintaining a stable airway can be challenging. Providing adequate gas exchange and then weaning from mechanical ventilation is fraught with difficulties. A thick layer of fatty tissue can make breath sounds very hard to hear. Chest x-rays can be poorly penetrated, thus assessment of pulmonary function sometimes will rely more on blood gas analysis, ventilatory pressures, amount, appearance culture, and sensitivity results of sputum, and tracheal suctioning.

Prior to extubation or full weaning from mechanical ventilation, the patient's ability to adequately take deep breaths should be assessed. Knowing whether the patient has a history of sleep apnea will be helpful in guiding this phase of pulmonary management. Optimizing pulmonary function during mechanical ventilation and weaning requires careful management. As weaning progresses, ventilatory support is reduced to allow greater patient participation in breathing. The patient's spontaneous breaths must be sufficient to provide a good tidal volume thus preventing or reducing atelectasis. Position changes while in bed are vital to help mobilize secretions and to improve gas exchange and reduce intra-pulmonary shunting. Weaning may be expedited by placing the patient in a semi-Fowler's position.[31,32] Many larger patients carry excessive weight in their abdominal region. When placed in a high-Fowler's position, the fatty tissue compresses against the diaphragm, therefore compromising respiratory function. Once hemodynamic stability is achieved, use of a chair specially designed for the obese patient is desirable. An oversized reclining wheelchair has been helpful in some critical care. Following extubation, increasing activity and encouraging Joe to cough and take deep breaths to clear secretions is critical. These activities serve to maintain adequate gas exchange and to reduce atelectasis. He should avoid both the supine and high-Fowler's positions as both place undue pressure on the diaphragm. Nasal CPAP (continuous positive airway pressure) can be helpful as an adjunct in the long-term management of OSA; however, post-extubation, many patients find this difficult to tolerate. BIPAP as a bridge after extubation and at night is especially helpful to prevent sleep apnea and hypoventilation.

During emergency intubation, it may be difficult to visualize anatomic landmarks, such as vocal cords, in the morbidly obese patient. The

Combitube (Mansfield, Massachusetts), an esophageal tracheal double lumen airway, is recognized by the American Heart Association and the American Society of Anesthesiologists as an alternative to the endotracheal tube when obesity-related technical difficulties arise.[33] Even in a nonemergency situation, airway management can be challenging. Standard tracheostomy tubes can be too short for use in the presence of a very thick neck. Some clinicians use an endotracheal tube. Others use the Rusch ultra tracheoflex 8mm or 9mm (Duluth, Georgia), a trach tube specially designed for the morbidly obese patient, or the Portex, a specially measured and ordered tracheostomy tube from Shiley (St. Louis, Missouri). Use of appropriate equipment can complement care, leading to safer and more effective care.

## MED-SURGICAL UNIT

Lack of appropriately sized equipment creates a multitude of care issues.[34] Numerous obesity-related complications are due to the inability to move patients adequately. During a prolonged hospitalization, difficulties in turning, transferring or ambulating patients may lead to immobility-related skin breakdown.[35] For example, pressure ulcers can occur in skin folds,

in areas where tubes and catheters have created prolonged pressure, or in any other area of the body that has been exposed to unrelieved pressure.[38] Pressure from side rails and arm rests not designed to accommodate an obese person can cause pressure ulcers on the patient's hips; this atypical skin breakdown can be minimized by using properly sized equipment. Oversized walkers, wheelchairs, commodes, bed frames, specialty mattresses, such as pressure relief or pressure reduction support surfaces, lateral rotation therapy, and lifts, can reduce or eliminate complications related to prolonged immobility.[37] Equipment designed to assist in moving, transferring, or lifting obese patients creates a setting more sensitive to the safety of the patient and members of the clinical team.

Psychologic issues of a more serious nature emerge at this time. Joe reported several instances of thinking he heard staff members discussing his weight in a degrading manner. He felt too weak to address that breach in privacy at the time, but was quite angry once he began to feel better. The clinicians reported that Joe seemed either passive and withdrawn or angry and acting out. It is not unusual for the patient to express anger or disappointment on admission to the med-surgical area. This may also be the time when patients express their desire to lose weight. Therefore, it becomes important for clinicians to recognize factors that prompt thoughts about behavior changes.

From birth, our behavior is aimed at doing what we believe will best satisfy one or more of our needs. By using information around them, babies learn what feels good and what feels bad, and how to satisfy their needs by obtaining what they need from others around them. All human beings carry this trait throughout life. This trait drives behavioral change and is an important consideration in helping patients reach the goals they establish for themselves. Glasser explains that the word motivation is largely misunderstood. Motivation must come from within; it is impossible to motivate another person. Therefore, clinicians are mistaken when they believe they can motivate the patient to change behavior. By saying, "My patient lacks motivation," clinicians are more likely expressing, "I am frustrated because I lack the power to control the patient." Control theory gives permission to clinicians to stop controlling and act collaboratively. The clinician's paternalistic responsibility is transformed

into a mutually responsive mentor:client relationship. However, an effective mentor provides sound information and realistic support that allows the client to take control of decision-making. This applies to all areas of chronic illness and other chronic conditions, including obesity. Clinicians who are interested in working with their larger clients in addressing issues of health promotion best serve the client when they understand what drives the individual to engage in or resist change.

## REHABILITATION

Following a long hospitalization, patients like Joe are often physically and emotionally exhausted. Caregivers fear injuring themselves and their patients. Even the most compassionate caregivers express concern in caring for larger, complex patients. Planning for appropriate rehabilitation care can be complicated.

Like Joe, some obese patients will have wounds in varying stages of healing. Because of diabetes and other comorbidities associated with obesity, the patient may have experienced delays in wound healing. A variety of types of skin injury can occur as a result of prolonged hospitalization. Pressure-related breakdown needs to be treat-

ed as such. The Agency for Healthcare Research and Quality has published guidelines for assessment, prevention, and treatment of pressure ulcers.[38,39]

Finally, mobility is critical in the rehabilitation patient. However, this can be especially challenging for patients who are emotionally discouraged, afraid of falling, or simply weak. Caregivers often hold the realistic fear of injuring themselves or their patients when they do not have access to size-appropriate equipment to achieve a task. Equipment specially designed for overweight patients is one option available to caregivers to make it easier and safer for them to perform patient activities. Specialized equipment is thought to facilitate patient rehabilitation and shorten the recovery period, while maintaining patient dignity.[40]

In planning care for obese patients, it may best serve the institution, caregivers, and patients to consider the value of a timely interdisciplinary team conference, which identifies appropriate equipment and adequate resources. Many of the more common, predictable, and costly complications can be prevented by an interdisciplinary team conference designed to identify early in the rehabilitation period what the patient's unique needs are. It is critical to

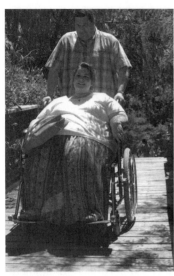

**In planning care for obese patients, it may best serve the institution, caregivers, and patients to consider the value of a timely interdisciplinary team conference, which identifies appropriate equipment and adequate resources.**

patient and caregiver safety to have appropriately sized equipment, for reasons described earlier. Resources within and outside the organization can be identified. This should also include staffing resources to help with the physical care of the patient. The purpose of the interdisciplinary team is to provide each discipline an opportunity to identify their specific goal for the patient, along with equipment and resources to meet these goals.

Typically, members of the interdisciplinary team would include the physician, physical therapist, nurse, occupational therapist, dietitian, respiratory therapist, pharmacist, and counselor, among others. Some rehabilitation settings include the patient and family members as part of the team because this tends to formalize the commitment between the patient, caregivers, and the rehabilitation plan. Physical therapists help the patient to transfer, ambulate, and otherwise increase activity and subsequently endurance. Goals set by occupational therapists often entail greater independence in activities of daily living. Bathing can be a difficult function for obese patients. Skin folds can cause special hygiene problems that the occupational therapist can creatively address with the patient. Nurses tend to collaborate with other disciplines to balance the patient's functional, emotional, physical, medical, and spiritual well being. Sharon Balters explains that the goal of the rehabilitation nurse is to establish a relationship based on trust while providing the patient with consistent feedback and coaching.[42]

Many overweight patients are actually undernourished, especially if nutrition was neglected during the acute episode.[43] The goal of the dietitian is likely to emphasize food choices within the context of health and well being, taking into account any co-existing diagnoses, such as diabetes. One of the goals of the respiratory therapist is to help the patient achieve an adequate level of rest. This is thought to be difficult for larger patients because of sleep apnea or OHS as described earlier.

Some medications are absorbed primarily in adipose tissue, while others in the muscle. The pharmacist can be instrumental in tailoring a medication plan unique to a patient who may have a higher percentage of body fat than most.[43] Psychologists or other counseling specialists can guide the patient in identifying behaviors that may interfere with a healthy lifestyle. Many larger patients may be depressed and withdrawn and may express feelings of helplessness and hopelessness, especially after a prolonged hospitalization. This discipline is skilled at encouraging patients to be more accepting of themselves and more active in meeting their emotional and physical needs.[44] Because of the range of skin injuries that can occur, the WOCN/ET can prove to be a valuable asset. Other disciplines may be added to the interdisciplinary team as indicated; however, the value of an interdisciplinary team is in its timing—the earlier the better, as this provides a way for caregivers to prevent some of those common complications associated with caring for larger patients.

## HOME CARE

The goals of discharge planning are to focus on ways to maximize the patient's physical and emotional transition toward independence in the home setting. In developing a plan of discharge care, the patient, family, and members of the interdisciplinary team should be involved.

The discharge planning needs of the obese patient are not unlike needs of the nonobese patient; yet a prolonged hospitalization or numerous comorbidities can intensify complexities. Not all obese patients will require special accommodation at home; however, patients who have limited mobility are likely to have special needs and therefore require special accommodation. In a recent study, nurses reported five specific challenges in the home care setting: equipment, reimbursement, access to resources, client motivation, and family/significant others support. The challenges cited most often involved specialized equipment issues.[45]

Many healthcare providers complain of the inability to turn, transfer, or lift heavier patients, which can lead to immobility-related concerns. Family members and caregivers may be at risk for injury when caring for the patient in the home, as fewer personnel are available to help. Oversized wheelchairs and walkers with greater weight limitations than standard equipment are readily available for purchase or rent in major medical supply centers. Both items promote independence and dignity. Equipment that nurses find most helpful in the home are the wheelchair, walker, commode, electronically controlled bed frame, support surface, and lift. When planning for oversized equipment in the home, consider weight limits, width, and electrical needs. In other words, does the patient have a sliding glass door or extra wide doorway through which equipment can be delivered? Can the equipment be dissembled, so that it can be delivered through a standard-sized doorway?

Community resources could include physical therapists, weight control counselors, and others. Written instructions for treatments, medication schedules, and follow-up appointments will be helpful in clarifying dates, times, and events for the patient.[45]

## CONCLUSION

Along with serious physical conditions, the obese patient brings very real emotional and social issues to the healthcare setting. Patients look to clinicians to provide safe and supportive expert care. Inclusion of specialists, including nursing peers, and specially designed equipment contribute to an interdisciplinary plan of care that provides the tools necessary to the clinician to delivery the safest, most sensitive, and appropriate care possible.

In developing a plan of care, the value of an interdisciplinary team cannot be overlooked. Because of the complex nature of caring for the obese patient, a variety of specialists, such as social workers, pulmonologists, physical therapists, dietitians, pharmacists, nurses, and others, including vendors, can offer valuable input. As we look to improve the quality of care for the larger patient in the healthcare setting, it will be increasingly important to ensure planning with appropriate resources.

## REFERENCES

1. Allison DB, Fontaine KR, Manson JE, et al. Annual deaths attributable to obesity in the United States. *J Am Med Assoc* 1999;282;1530–8.
2. Gallagher S, Langlois C, Spacht D, et al. Preplanning protocols for skin and wound care in obese patients. *Adv Skin Wound Care* 2004;17(8):436–43.
3. Gallagher S. Shedding weight with bariatric surgery. *Nursing* 2004;34:58–64.
4. Maiman LA, Wang VL, Becker MH, et al. Attitudes toward obesity and the obese among professionals. *J*

*Am Diet Assoc* 1992;74:331–6.

5. Segal-Isaacson C-J. American attitudes toward body fatness. *Nurs Pract* 1996;21:9–13.

6. Gallagher SM. Meeting the needs of the obese patient. *AJN* 1996;96 supp 1s–12s.

7. Kramer K, Gallagher S. WOC nurses as advocates for patients who are morbidly obese: A case study promoting use of bariatric beds. *J WOCN* 2004;31:276–81.

8. Gallagher S. Understanding compassion, sensitivity, and the obese patient. *Bariatric Times* 2004;1(1):4–8.

9. Goodell TT. The obese trauma patient: Treatment strategies. *J Trauma Nurs* 1996;3:36.

10. Gallagher SM. Caring for obese patients. *Nursing* 1998;28:32hn1–32hn3.

11. Maxwell MH. Errors in blood-pressure measurement due to incorrect cuff size in obese patients. *Lancet* 1982;2:33–6

12. Lachet MF, Owen JW, Ebel MD. Caring for the morbidly obese pregnant woman. *MCN* 1995;20:101–6.

13. Warner WA, Garrett LP. The obese patient and anesthesia. *J Am Med Assoc* 1968;205:92–3.

14. Catenacci AJ, Anderson JD, Boersma D. Anesthetic hazards of obesity. *J Am Med Assoc* 1961;175:657–65.

15. Gould AB Jr. Effects of obesity on respiratory complications following general anesthesia. *Anesth Analg* 1962;41:448–52.

16. Vaughn RN. Anesthesia and the Obese Patient. In: Brown BR Jr. (ed). *Contemporary Anesthesia Practice*. Philadelphia, PA: FA Davis Co., 1982.

18. Postlewait RW, Johnson WD. Complications following surgery for duodenal ulcers in obese patients. *Arch Surg* 1972;105:438–40.

19. Shinohara E, Kihara S, Yamashita S, et al. Visceral fat accumulation as an important risk factor for obesity sleep apnea syndrome in obese subjects. *J Int Med* 1997;24:11–18.

20. Diagnostic Classification Steering Committee of the American Sleep Disorders Association. The Classification of Sleep Disorders—Revised: Diagnostic and Coding Manual. Rochester, MN: Davies Printing Company, 1997.

21. Gleason JM. Obese hypoventilation syndrome. *Crit Care Nurse* 1987;7(6):74–8.

22. Shinohara E, Kihara S, Yamashita S, et al. Visceral fat accumulation as an important risk factor for obesity sleep apnea syndrome in obese subjects. *J Int Med* 1997;24:11–18.

23. Loube DI, Loube AA, Mitler MM. Weight loss for obstructive sleep apnea: The optimal therapy for obese patients. *J Am Diet Assoc* 1994;94:1291–4.

24. Kaltman AJ, Goldring RM. Role of circulatory congestion in cardiorespiratory failure in obesity. *Am J Med* 1976;60:645–53.

25. Langerstrand L, Rossner S. Effects of weight loss on pulmonary function in obese men with obstructive sleep apnea syndrome. *J Intern Med* 1993;234:245–7.

26. AARC Clinical Practice Guidelines. Metabolic measurement using indirect calorimetry during mechanical ventilation. *Resp Care* 1994;39:1170–5.

27. Salvi RJ. Metabolic monitoring. *Advances for Managers of Respiratory Care* 1997;3:40–42.

28. Gallagher SM. Meeting the needs of the obese patient. *AJN* 1996;96(supp1):1s–12s.

29. Shikora SA. Enteral feeding tube placement in obese patients: Consideration for nutritional support. *Nutrition in Clinical Practice* 1997;12:9s–13s.

30. Gallagher SM. Morbid obesity: A chronic disease with an impact on wounds and related problems. *Ostomy Wound Manage* 1997;43:18–27.

31. Gallagher SM. Morbid obesity: A chronic disease with an impact on wounds and related problems. *Ostomy Wound Manage* 1997;43:18–27.

32. Carpenter R, Burns SM, Egloff MB, et al. Effects of body position on spontaneous respiratory rate and tidal volume in patients with obesity, abdominal distention, and ascites. *J Crit Care* 1994;3:102–6.

33. Lasater-Erhad M. The effect of body position on arterial oxygen saturation. *Crit Care Nurs* 1995;15:31–6.

34. Banyai M, Falger S, Roggla M, et al. Emergency intubation with the Combitube in a grossly obese patient with bull neck. *Resusc* 1993;26:271–6.

35. Gallagher S, Arzouman J, Lacovara J, et al. Criteria-based protocols and the obese patient: Planning care for a high-risk population.

*Ostomy Wound Manage* 2004;50:32–44.

36. Gallagher SM. Morbid obesity: A chronic condition with an impact on wounds and wound problems. *Ostomy Wound Manage* 1997;43:18–27.

37. Gallagher SM. Meeting the needs of the obese patient. *AJN* 1996;96:1s–12s.

38. Gallagher SM. Tailoring care for obese patients. *RN* 1999;62:43–8.

39. Preventing Pressure Ulcers Guideline Panel. *Preventing Pressure Ulcers. Clinical Practice Guideline Number 4.* Rockville, MD: Agency for Health Care Policy and Research, Public Health Service, US Department of Health and Human Services; May 1992. AHCPR Publication No.92-0048.

40. Treatment of Pressure Ulcers Guideline Panel. *Treatment of Pressure Ulcers. Clinical Practice Guideline Number 15.* Rockville, MD: Agency for Health Care Policy and Research, Public Health Service, US Department of Health and Human Services; December 1994. AHCPR Publication No.95-0652

41. Gallagher SM. Caring for the overweight patient in acute care setting. *J Healthcare Safety Compliance Infection Control* 2000;4:379–82.

42. Balters S. Reclaiming lives. *Team Rehab.*1998;Nov.

43. Gallagher SM. Morbid obesity: A chronic condition with an impact on wounds and wound problems. *Ostomy Wound Manage* 1997;43:18–27.

44. Gallagher SM. Tailoring care for obese patients. *RN* 1999;62:43–50.

45. Balters S. Reclaiming lives. *Team Rehab* November 1998.

46. Gallagher SM. Needs of the homebound morbidly obese patient: A descriptive survey of home health nurses. *Ostomy Wound Manage* 1998;44:23–9.

**13**

# Caregiver Injury

**S**afety specialists, insurance carriers, administrators, caregivers, and consumers are increasingly aware that healthcare is fast becoming one of the most dangerous jobs in the US. Injuries are reaching epidemic levels. The Occupational Safety and Health Administration (OSHA) named ergonomics, especially in healthcare, as a top priority.[1]

Additionally, the Joint Commission on Accreditation of Healthcare Organizations (JCAHCO) surveyors is reportedly taking greater interest in caregiver and patient issues related to lifting and transferring. Hospitals report that surveyors are asking about preventive measures taken for the most frequent and/or costly injuries. This emerging interest is likely due to the increased economic and noneconomic costs of injury.[2] For example, caregivers suffer injury and possible disability with subsequent loss of wages, function, and even earning power. Additionally, caregivers are likely to suffer emotional pain. Patient falls can be costly to healthcare organizations, as they can be a source of litigation, pain, stress, and increased length of stay with inadequate reimbursement. According to the Bureau of Labor and Statistics, health-care workers are at particular risk for caregiver injury. The health-related jobs at greatest risk are nurse assistants, licensed vocational nurses (LVN), registered nurses (RN), radiology technicians, and physical therapists. Not surprising, the leaders of all industries in lost workdays due to back injuries are hospitals.[3]

Although most of the back injuries experienced by healthcare professionals have been thought to be cumulative and not resulting from a single incident, recent research suggests that back pain and other work-related musculoskeletal injures may in fact be caused not only by cumulative trauma to the spine and related structures but might also be due to a single traumatic event, such as a fall. Other factors identified as causes of back pain and other work-related musculoskeletal injures are genetics, age, poor physical condition, obesity, poor posture, tension, emotional stress, cigarette smoking, or bending, standing, sitting, or lifting improperly.

More than half of strains and sprains are attributed to manual lifting tasks that are

## THE STORY OF ANN

**A**nn is a 43-year-old registered nurse. She has worked in intensive care for 15 of her 20 years as a nurse. Fifteen months ago, while manually lifting a critically ill patient, she was overwhelmed with pain and numbness. She had sustained a significant back injury, yet attempted to continue to work for 13 more months until she could no longer focus on her work because of the massive doses of medication that were needed to control her pain and other emerging symptoms. Ann's story illustrates the noneconomic implications in caregiver injury, and reflects the meaning of quality of life when a caregiver injury occurs.

Ann has explained that she is really angry about her situation. She also stresses that this is not an economic issue for her, but is something much bigger. First of all, there are role changes that must be dealt with, as she is no longer employable. So much of our self esteem and self image are reflected in our work, and when asked, "What do you do?" her response is, "I'm unemployed."

Ann also shared that her years of education, training, and experience are now unimportant or meaningless in a work-oriented culture. "I'm not asked to use my brain any more, and it's killing me." She explains that, "No part of my life is unaffected!"

In addition to the issues of self-esteem, there are actual physical issues with which she never imagined she would need to face. First of all, consider the family's shock when it was discovered that she could no longer rock climb, hike, or mountain bike with them. The vehicle she had driven for three years needed to be replaced because she could no longer get into it comfortably. "I can't shop, I can't dress myself comfortably...and imagine the idea of sex when the back pain is constant." Ann explains that life revolves around her back and that this is trying for her friends and family.

"The only member of my family who is happy with me anymore is my dog, because the only activity I can do comfortably is walk briskly. It's really a pathetic existence—I would not wish this on anyone."

performed while assisting dependent patients with their mobility needs. Injuries that result from manual lifting and transferring of patients are among the most frequent causes of caregiver injuries. These and other patient care tasks are becoming increasingly more difficult for patient care[4] providers as the patient population changes. Patient size, weight, and acuity, along with limited facility resources (e.g., inadequate equipment and personnel) affect incidence of caregiver injury.[5]

The implication for caregivers is that turning, lifting, and repositioning very dependent heavier patients can predispose caregivers to physical injury. Additionally, failure to provide adequate patient activity and mobility leads to issues of patient safety.[6] This article describes caregiver injury as it impacts bariatric patients, clinicians, and clinical care.

Ergonomics is also described, and the role of the ergonomist is described as a resource to patient care providers. The emotional and economic aspects of injury are included. A variety of strategies are available to reduce or prevent caregiver injury and to promote patient safety. This article includes discussion of transfer/lift teams, appropriate equipment, and criteria-based protocols. The philosophy of continuous quality improvement is presented as a model for change. Techniques for mobility are also described.

## ERGONOMICS

Ergonomics is the art and science that considers the physical stress and environmental factors influencing caregiver safety and productivity. An ergonomist might serve as a resource to the caregiver to assess his or her work environment and habits and identify and make recommendations to reduce potential risk factors and hazards.

Recommendations include keeping necessary objects within reach, minimizing the amount of contact stressors or repetitious tasks, maintaining a neutral position, and taking care to perform activities at a height that prevents over-reaching or bending. The ergonomist might suggest ways to minimize mental or physical fatigue and create a comfortable environment, thus ensuring a role in the patient care team.[7]

## COSTS OF INJURY

A number of studies reveal the increasing incidence, cost, and number of caregiver injury claims associated with patient care. To date, low back pain, which affects men and women and is most common in those between the ages of 25 and 45, is the leading cause of job-related injury and disability. For example, 89 percent of back injury claims filed by hospitals are related to patient handling, and the direct costs associated with these injuries exceed $15,000 per claim.

Workers' compensation back injuries cost 255 percent more than non-work–related back injuries, and hospitalization is twice as likely for these individuals.

About 80 percent of adults are estimated to experience a back injury in their lifetime, and about 10 percent will suffer re-injury. Back injuries are cited as the most common reason for absenteeism in the general workplace, second only to the common cold. In fact, in 2001, there were 121,562 new back injury claims, and the cost related to those back injury claims was $52 million. There were almost 60,000 ongoing claims, and the costs associated with those claims reached nearly $300 million.[7] Despite ongoing interest and concern with back-related injuries, most recently injuries to the neck and shoulders are on the rise. Some suggest this is due to lateral transfer activities and the heavier patient (See: The Danger of Lateral Transfer).[5]

It is important to recognize that the economic costs are only a portion of the real cost of occupational injuries. Injured caregivers are faced with time lost from work, emotional and physical distress, job and career changes, and role changes at home (See: The Story of Ann). There are also hidden costs for the organization, such as lost revenue due to a loss in productivity, decreased employee retention, costly orientation of new staff, diminished staff morale, and added administrative time for investigation and paperwork.

When hospitalized, clinicians should recognize that most very dependent patients are at risk for certain hazards of immobility. When physically dependent, the patient is more inclined to develop costly complications and a lengthier hospitalization. Common immobility-related complications include skin breakdown, pulmonary concerns, and pain management. Immobility can lead to feelings of powerlessness. Mobilizing the patient early and safely can reduce some of these immobility-related complications of hospitalization, and yet fear of caregiver injury threatens these activities.

## FEAR OF CAREGIVER INJURY

In addition to the patient care hazards of immobility, there can be hazards to caregivers when mobilizing the very weak, larger, dependent patient. Even the most compassionate caregiver's attitude and intervention can be influenced by the realistic fear of physical injury. Consider the numerous court cases involving injured registered nurses

and other caregivers and their inability to provide care that entails lifting or transferring. Hospitals are not legally mandated to ensure assistance to the caregiver who is providing these activities. In addition, this failure to accommodate the needs of an injured caregiver further perpetuates the potential for injuring other healthcare workers. In other words, when injured caregivers are removed from their roles, others are added as replacements. The process for care does not change, only the people—the noninjured are substituted for the injured. This problem not only affects the injured but the noninjured, or those who are likely to be injured in the future. This is a mounting healthcare concern fueling the fear of injury.

## THE PATIENT AT RISK

Physical pain and the fear of falling pose special risks. Falls pose a serious risk for hospitalized patients, and are typically thought to be a problem of the elderly population. However, falls are increasingly common among heavier, sicker, or physically dependent patients, regardless of age. And when a large, heavy patient does fall, the consequences can be profound for the patient and caregiver (See: The Obese Patient). Falls impact patients, care-

givers, and organizations. Patient falls are extremely costly in terms of injury and disability with a subsequent impairment of function and quality of life for the patient. Even patients who are able to maintain the highest level of functioning and independence at home may be compromised upon entering the hospital environment. For example, the home environment may be modified to allow for the patient's size, strength, and unique physical needs. There may be wide pathways through rooms with handrails or heavy furniture that the patient may use for balance. The patient and/or caregiver may have devised certain workable routines for daily activities, such as bathing, toileting, and exercise. However, in the hospital, the patient is presented with equipment that does not suit his or her physical needs, preventing safe activity and mobility. Most furnishings in the hospital environment are on wheels, and this is not safe or adequate to support a dependent person attempting to transfer in and out of a bed or chair, or to ambulate around the room or restroom.

The patient may be in a weakened condition with decreased balance or function due to illness, medication, pain, immobility, or dietary changes associated with a hospital admission. Often the obese patient is not only fearful of falling and incurring injury to him- or herself, but also of falling on or otherwise causing injury to a caregiver.

Pain can interfere with patient mobility for physiologic and psychological reasons. In most cultures, pain serves as a warning that something is wrong. Patients experiencing pain often respond with reluctance to move or participate in activity and mobility. The patient may be resistant to repositioning, transfers, or other activity because of sustained discomfort. Often this reluctance is misinterpreted as nonadherent or health-defeating behavior. Pain and fear both can place the patient at risk for dependence, thus placing the caregiver at risk for injury.

## ADDRESSING CAREGIVER INJURY

An interdisciplinary approach that is comprised of clinical experts, equipment, and education is thought to best serve the goal of caregiver health and safety. Many hospitals have formally or informally adopted the goal of a physical therapy/occupational therapy (PT/OT) assessment of the patient's functional status within eight hours of admission. PT/OT staff can then provide caregiver orientation to include use of any specialized equip-

### DANGERS OF THE LATERAL TRANSFER

**H**istorically, back injuries have been the most common type of injury among healthcare workers. However, some contend this is changing as the population changes. Sara is an experienced radiology technologist who cares for dozens of patients every day. She reports that her responsibilities include reassuring patients, preparing and performing radiologic procedures, and positioning patients on the radiology table. The weight limit of the radiology table is 375 pounds; therefore, she does not have opportunity to work with severely obese patients. Yet due to the rising number of larger patients who require assistance with lateral transfers, she has increasingly experienced neck and shoulder pain.

Sara explains that as she discusses her condition with other clinicians, she discovered her situation is not unique. Lateral transfers are a growing concern for two reasons. Not only does this activity pose a threat to caregivers, but this action can lead to shearing injury, which contributes to serious skin and tissue damage among immobile or dependent patients. After much debate and consideration, Sara was asked to present her thoughts on her shoulder and neck injury, along with ideas for preventing the dangers of lateral transfers not only to herself but to the patient as well.

A growing number of hospitals and clinics have introduced an air displacement system that works by release of low pressure air through perforated chambers. This lateral transfer device works like the Hover Craft, a water and land craft that had military indications early in the twentieth century. Lateral air transfer technology provides for lateral transfers of patients up to 1,000 pounds, with the assistance of one to two caregivers. When the device is inflated, the displaced air actually lifts the patient through the perforated underside, reducing friction and encouraging movement with the slightest effort. This and other innovative products are available to encourage patient safety and mobility, while protecting caregivers like Sara from injury.

ment or mobility techniques.

Regularly scheduled inservice/orientation to repeat/reinforce previous instruction should include use of equipment and specific mobility techniques. All staff should be educated on proper techniques for moving the dependent

patient. A key point is to ensure that the number of personnel assisting the patient is adequate/appropriate for the task. More helpers may not always ensure a higher degree of safety. Adequate personnel coupled with adequate equipment may serve as the best combination for safety.

In addition to training on use of equipment, the PT/OT and/or ergonomist can be instrumental in teaching skills, such as transferring—which is thought to be a serious threat to caregivers if performed improperly. The degree of difficulty in transferring patients will depend on the functional status of the patient. In other words, not every patient will pose a risk of injury. However, fear, pain, weakness, dependence, obesity, or a low level of cooperation will pose such risk.

Some tasks are more difficult than others. For example, one of the most frequent and difficult tasks to accomplish is the bed to chair transfer. The challenge of this task varies depending on how physically dependent the patient is. With a totally dependent patient, in order to have access to the patient, the caregiver must reach across the bed. This is especially true in the case of caring for larger patients in wider beds. The bed serves as an obstacle. The caregiver probably will not be able to bend his or her knees because he or she is leaning up against the bed. If the patient needs to be physically lifted, the weight of the load involved in the lift is unacceptable for a typical caregiv-

er. In addition, the transfer into a chair requires moving the patient to a different height level; some carrying is usually involved. Therefore, the risk factors of this particular task include reaching, lifting a load using suboptimal lifting postures, and carrying a load a distance. These types of transfers have traditionally been identified as high-risk activities.

The PT/OT or ergonomist holds special knowledge in understanding and selecting products designed for transferring patients. In using lift systems, the lift must be easily maneuverable and clear in operational instructions. Make sure the lift maintains balance when the patient is seated in the sling. The lift should be constructed so that it is able to lift a patient up off the floor if necessary. If the patient can bear weight, use a standard-assist lift and make sure the knee and foot supports are adjustable. For lateral transfers, consider a slide board, roll board, seated transfer boards, or air-filled transfer devices. In all products, consider both weight limit and width accommodation.[8]

Although patient handling techniques may differ from patient to patient, some general principles for care exist. Assess the patient's mental and physical abilities

to participate in the transfer task, including weight-bearing status. Make sure footwear and clothing are appropriate for the transfer. Ensure personal privacy by providing adequately sized gowns. Know before the transfer what equipment is necessary, secure the equipment, and know the amount of assistance needed. Identify all barriers, such as IV tubes and catheters, that interfere with movement. Instruct the patient clearly, providing sufficient time for feedback to ensure the patient has fully understood the directions. Take the opportunity to demonstrate the transfer if necessary. Do not grasp the patient's arm or clothing; instead use a safety belt or sheet on the patient. The caregiver's body should be positioned closely to the patient in order to safely guard or lead the patient throughout the transfer. Transfer the patient to his or her stronger side. Ensure there is help throughout the activity. Once the transfer is complete, position the patient so that he or she is comfortable and stable, and place essential objects in the patient's safe reach.[9]

Organizations best serve their employees and their patients, especially the weak and immobile obese patient, when issues concerning patient safety and caregiver injury are addressed; however, most agree that this is slowly and inconsistently forthcoming.

## MAKING CHANGES

Organizations seek a number of creative ways to prevent caregiver injury. Of these, transfer teams, appropriate equipment and criteria-based protocols have been useful in achieving this goal.

Transfer teams, sometimes called lift teams, are thought to reduce or prevent caregiver injury in some settings. For instance, in the early 1990s, during an organization-wide nursing shortage, one hospital discovered a significant increase in the number of nursing injuries. Coincidentally, there was a significant increase in workers' compensation and operation costs. Hospital staff members from a variety of disciplines collaborated to create a task force to address the nursing injury issue. The task force discovered the work of William Charney, who had developed the concept of a lift team that had been successful in other organizations that were addressing similar challenges. Charney's lift team became the model to serve as part of the injury management team. His research on the concept as a holistic approach to nursing injury prevention has proven successful when confronting lost time injuries related to nurses and lifting patients.

The lift team comprises individuals who have been screened and found to be at low risk for injury. Members are carefully trained to perform patient lifting and transferring activities. Team members are provided with patient handling equipment and are skilled in using the equipment to perform strenuous patient-handling tasks. The current trend is to incorporate a stronger education, training, and consultative component, which supports nurses and others to perform safer mobility activities.

Lift team intervention reduces the frequency and severity of nursing injuries that result from patient handling. The lift team has become an accepted adjunct to the patient care team. The lift team intervention is believed to have improved nursing morale and patient satisfaction with regard to patient handling tasks. Lift team intervention programs do prevent work-related injuries and should be considered by patient institutions.

Criteria-based protocols for use of specially designed equipment are intended to ensure more appropriate, timely, and cost-sensitive use of equipment. Performance improvement (PI) teams offer a resource to develop and implement appropriate policies and resources for equipment needs.

Implementing changes to better manage the unique care issues for the weak patient can be challenging for caregivers. The initial cost of any change is often viewed as an obstacle. Without a thorough understanding of the cost incurred in caregiver injury and the prolonged hospitalization of the patient, it may be difficult to economically justify introduction of specialized equipment, which very well may not be reimbursed by third party payers.

Most agree that in the healthcare delivery market, a successful organization must remain profitable while maintaining or improving the quality of its services. JCAHCO recognizes the numerous barriers to change and has adopted the philosophy of continuous quality improvement (CQI) as a cornerstone for change, and the management principles of CQI continue to gain acceptance in the healthcare industry. Performance improvement is a recent innovation that utilizes these principles of CQI in making changes in health organizations.

A PI team, based on the principles of CQI, seeks to make changes that improve the therapeutic, cost, and satisfaction outcomes associated with patient care. Decisions need to be made by those individuals closest to the patient and be customer-focused, and change must continue to be ongoing. A task force could include a physical therapist, occupational health coordinator, risk manager, safety specialist, ergonomist, front-line caregiver, and administrator. Vendors are also valuable in this process because they are able to partner with hospitals that are looking for equipment that could be tailored to better meet the needs of caregivers. These quality-based efforts can be unit-based or house-wide. Regardless, they are important to consider in that they can more accurately establish the actual needs of the organizations as they seek to reduce or prevent caregiver injury.

## A LOOK TO THE FUTURE

Increases in the number of very ill, very dependent patients tremendously affects healthcare delivery. This increasing prevalence will impact acute care and may influence the frequency of admission as well as the level of care that patients require when hospitalized. Clinicians best serve the needs of the patient when policies and protocols are in place to care for the patient. Continued use of interdisciplinary teams is essential to more fully understand the interdepartmental impact of caring for overweight

### THE OBESE PATIENT

Although attempts to reduce body weight are common among Americans, the prevalence of obesity has continued to increase since the 1980s. Considering that more than 67 percent of US adults are overweight, it is likely that issues of caring for the overweight patient will continue. In fact, what is even more concerning is that not only has the percentage of adult obese Americans increased, but the number of overweight children has doubled. And even though some overweight people are able to lose some of their body weight, a majority regain that weight within five years. Therefore, attention to ensuring caregiver safety lies in part in addressing care of larger, heavier patients.

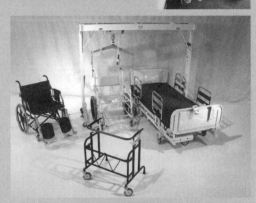

Heavy-duty walkers, which accommodate patients weighing from 350 to 1,000 pounds, make it easier to safely assist in ambulating heavy, weak patients. Beds, support surfaces, and wheelchairs that support up to 1,000 pounds are also available. In addition, a number of lift designs are available to safely mobilize the very large patient. Providing equipment specially designed for the bariatric patient is important for reducing work-related back injuries among caregivers and thus lowering the risk of related patient injuries.

Healthcare facilities must have a plan in place to care for the special needs of the weak, obese patient. Preplanning with manufacturers and vendors to provide restorative equipment for the deconditioned obese patient is essential. Institutional policies and procedures to obtain transportation and transfer devices, bed frames and support surfaces, wheelchairs, walkers, and commodes or furniture must be available.

A key point is to ensure that the number of personnel assisting the patient is adequate for the task. Additionally, more helpers may not ensure a higher degree of safety. Adequate personnel coupled with proper equipment and education may serve as the best combination for safety!

patients in the acute care setting. Furthermore, manufacturers and vendors need clinical input in order to more fully understand the unique equipment needs of the patient. Clinicians best serve their patients when they are able to partner with the industry to creatively seek solutions to the challenges described.

## CONCLUSION

Perhaps insufficient attention to issues of immobility, patient safety, and caregiver injury is more a product of inadequate identification of those patients who pose risks. The patient may or may not be identified by an admitting diagnosis and /or list of clinical problems. Caregivers and patients are best served when the patient is properly identified and preplanning begins before admission to the hospital.

Managing the complex needs of today's patient can be time consuming and costly.[10] Solutions to this industry-wide problem of caregiver injury are not simple. Collaborative task forces are in the best position to understand the issues more fully, as each department is affected in a unique yet very important manner. A number of solutions may exist; however, transfer teams and use of appropriate equipment supported by criteria-based protocols is one strategy. Quality improvement theories may be helpful to develop and sustain these efforts to reduce or prevent caregiver injury. The challenge to hospitals and caregivers is that all these changes must be done in a growing climate where profit and reductions outweigh safety. Preplanning care is designed to control costs by preventing caregiver injury and promoting patient safety. An interdisciplinary approach is likely to best serve the needs of the patient, caregivers, and the institution.

## REFERENCES

1. *Back disorders and injuries.* Occupational Safety and Health Administration (OSHA). Available at: www.osha.org. Access date: November 2004.
2. Back Injury Prevention. Available at: www.premierinc.com/all/safety/resources/back_injury/index.html. Access date: November 2004.
3. Bielecki JT. Back injuries in health-care workers. *Occupational Health Tracker: Journal of Trends and Strategies for Occupational Health Professionals* 2002;5:1–4.
4. Charney W, Hudson MA (eds). *Back Injury Among Healthcare Workers.* New York, NY: Lewis Press, 2004.
5. Gallagher S. Caring for the overweight patient in the acute care setting: addressing caregiver injury. *J Healthcare Safety Compliance Infection Control* 2000;4:379–82.
6. Gallagher S. Obesity: Considering mobility, patient safety, and caregiver injury. In: Charney W, Hudson MA (eds). *Back Injury Among Healthcare Workers.* New York, NY: Lewis Press, 2004.
7. OSHA announces comprehensive plan to reduce ergonomic injuries. *Occupational Safety and Health Administration* (OSHA). Available at: www.osha.org. Access date: June, 2004.
8. Patient lift and transfer resources. *Reducing Musculoskeletal Injuries in Patient Care.* Available at: www.patientsafetycenter.com/safe. Access date: November, 2004.
9. Pierson FM, Fairchild SL. *Principles and Techniques of Patient Care.* Philadelphia, PA: WB Saunders, 2002.
10. U.S. Department of Labor, Bureau of Labor Statistics, 2000. Available at: www.bls.gov. Access date: June, 2004.

# Outcomes in Bariatric Care

**E**ach day healthcare providers are tracking hundreds of different methods of delivering care. Projects, policies, and procedures are scrutinized daily. Outcome initiatives have become important to the long-term success of healthcare organizations. A few well chosen outcome projects can be critical to safe patient care, and especially bariatric patient care.[1]

The outcome movement as we know it today grew out of the quality improvement effort first described formally by W. Edwards Deming. However, outcomes have been measured before the time of Florence Nightingale.[2] Mortality and morbidity, length of stay, adverse nosocomial events, and other quality indicators are likely opportunities for improvement.[3] This movement is gaining interest for many reasons. The rise in healthcare costs is one factor that has increased provider, payer, and patient interest in therapeutic, satisfaction, and financial outcomes. It has been over a decade since Ellwood offered a framework and vision for implementing health-related outcomes management programs.

A number of factors have opened the doors to outcome research as we know it today. Rising healthcare costs have increased provider, payer, and patient interests in therapeutic, satisfaction, and financial outcomes. An overriding healthcare concern is enhancing quality while providing services in an efficient and cost-effective manner.[4] Outcomes are the key to understanding the effectiveness of cost-sensitive patient care.[5] Outcomes by definition are the end result of care, or a measurable change in the patient's health status or behavior because of a well-defined intervention.[6]

The explosion of computer hardware and software that occurred in the 1980s has made measurement of financial outcomes easily aggregated and measurable by providers. Surprisingly, longitudinal therapeutic and satisfaction outcomes have not been so forthcoming.[7]

## A HISTORICAL PERSPECTIVE

Deming championed revolutionary concepts designed to improve management strategies and productivity outcomes. His work was initially pioneered in industry and later in healthcare and a

---

**IDEAS ON OUTCOME OPPORTUNITIES[10]**

- **Measures can be unit-based or extend throughout the organization**
- **Measures must relate to the organization's strategic plan**
- **Measures should be based on internal and external influences**
- **Measures should empower employees**
- **Review of the measures should be systematic**

---

number of other services. He believed that customers and employees should be involved in an ongoing process designed to improve quality, cost-efficiency, and customer satisfaction.[8] Deming posed a philosophy of quality improvement, and clinicians are charged with operationalizing this philosophy. Although his philosophy hasn't changed, the models currently used in healthcare settings continue to evolve. It has been a decade since Paul Ellwood provided a framework and a vision for implementing outcomes management programs. Although progress has been made since that time, the number of documented improvements in clinical or therapeutic outcomes and satisfaction outcomes has been moderate primarily because health systems have focused largely on cost containment.

But now that valid and reliable tools and sophisticated information systems are available to quantify important aspects of health and well being from the patient's

perspective, it is expected that progress in identifying, measuring, and managing patient outcomes will lead to objective improvement.

## DEFINING OUTCOMES

Outcomes by definition are a means to provide quantitative documentation that a change in clinical practice makes a difference in a cost, clinical, or satisfaction outcome. Examples of outcome research, pertaining to obesity, are presented in three domains: caring for the individual, institutionally specific (e.g., criteria-based protocol or system-wide [public policy]), which could drive reimbursement policies. Within those domains, change occurs to address specific high cost, high frequency clinical problems across practice settings. Clinicians in home, hospital, outpatient, and long-term care have concerns about caring for the very large patient. Difficulties in turning, transferring, or ambulating patients can lead to immobility-related outliers. For example, pressure ulcers can occur in patients who are very heavy and difficult to turn. Pressure ulcers can occur in skin folds, in areas where tubes and catheters have created prolonged pressure, or any other area of the body that has been exposed to unrelieved pressure. In addition to immobility-related skin breakdown, other kinds of skin injury can occur. Obstructive respiratory consequences can lead to costly, lengthy hospitalization. Chronic, acute, or emotional pain can also affect outcomes, as do inappropriate access to equipment. Fear of caregiver injury is yet another threat to patient care. Consider the patient with a tracheostomy or a colostomy. For example, tracheostomy care can pose a challenge postoperatively, not only because of the tracheostomy, but because of the large surgical wound created to locate the trachea. Additionally, tracheostomy ties may pose a challenge. Narrow cloth ties designed to secure the tracheostomy tube could burrow into skin folds within the soft tissue, causing pressure necrosis. To complicate matters, perspiration and secretions in the surrounding area could lead to an increased bacterial load, which threatens wound healing. An introduction of wider tracheostomy tube holders could be a

simple, yet very cost-effective way of securing the tracheostomy tube. But without evidence to that extent, it is difficult for many clinicians to justify additional costs.

Colostomy care can be challenging because of the presence of skin folds, irregularities in the contour of the abdomen, or the presence of a large abdominal pannus. The inability to maintain a good seal between the colostomy pouch and the skin can result in denuded skin and costly pouch changes. Perhaps a preoperative visit by a wound, ostomy, continence nurse (WOCN) to mark the stoma placement can guide the surgeon to the best location on the patient's irregularly contoured abdomen, which ultimately may reduce costs and increase patient satisfaction.

Obstructive respiratory problems can lead to longer and more costly admissions. Immobility may lead to respiratory problem. On the other hand, obstructive diseases may lead to respiratory failure and consequently a prolonged hospitalization.

Obese patients often have chronic pain commonly due to osteoarthritis of the knees, hips, or shoulders.

Emotional pain is not unusual, especially among patients who have been admitted to acute or long-term care facilities that are not adequately equipped or prepared to handle very large patients. Disrespectful comments, discussion, and otherwise unprofessional behaviors can affect the emotional well-being of the patient. Acute pain is often the result of surgery, procedures, treatments, or simply uncomfortable surroundings. Pain is thought to interfere with rehabilitation and length of stay.

Hesitation on the part of the caregiver to provide care simply because of the fear of injury is a threat to patient care and ultimately outcomes. Each of these examples provided could interfere with the patient's progress, but these issues are only a few. Opportunities for improvement are based largely on the unique needs of the facility. The challenge to clinicians is to recognize opportunities as they present themselves, and to familiarize themselves with the tools necessary to begin the process of improvement. Organizational-based protocols are often used to reduce

## UNDERSTANDING LONG-TERM RESEARCH

Long-term outcome research on the success of bariatric surgery extends back about 15 years. Although a comprehensive approach to care was encouraged at that time, the level of emphasis that currently exists on the psychology of this procedure, the importance of nutritional education, and the importance of behavioral modification was not present. It remains to be seen in future research what these preoperative improvements provide in the years to come. In the meantime, making sure that patients have had a professional and thorough preoperative psychological evaluation adds dimensions to the patient's total care that otherwise would not be present. Creating an outcome project that specifically addresses the value of an interdisciplinary approach continues to offer clinicians at all levels an opportunity to describe the most effective strategies in bariatric care.

the cost of common and predictable complications among certain groups of patients.

Most researchers agree that the three categories of outcomes are therapeutic, cost, or satisfaction outcomes. Unfortunately, outcomes are sometimes regarded in one domain more than another. For example, the focus may be only on cost outcomes, when in fact those of a therapeutic or satisfaction nature can be just as meaningful. All three are important and are probably more closely related than not.

By definition, therapeutic or clinical outcomes are concerned with improving the quality of treatments or procedures around patient care. Therapeutic outcomes are designed to improve clinical parameters or improve the patient's physical being. Cost outcomes, sometimes called financial or economic outcomes, look at reducing the costs of delivering care without an adverse impact on quality. Satisfaction outcomes, sometimes referred to as humanistic or quality of life outcomes, examine those changes that are likely to improve the patient or family's level of satisfaction with care, quality of life, or adaptation to illness.

Outcome efforts comprise the following three steps: outcome identification, outcome measurement, and outcome management. In the first step of outcome identification, the clinician needs to define a specific target population, seek measurable results, identify a goal that is attainable, and recognize time and resource limitations. In this first step, the clinician

must formulate an appropriate question. For example, the question, "What is the percentage of bariatric patients that develop complications postoperatively?" is not appropriate because it is too vague to establish a measurable criterion for improvement. Instead one might ask, "What percent of patients with a body mass index (BMI) of 45 to 55, who have surgery lasting longer than three hours develop skin injury within the first three postoperative days?" or "What effect does introduction of a lift/transfer system have on caregiver injury when caring for a patient with a BMI greater than 45?" or "What effect does preoperative stoma placement marking have on postoperative skin care for patients having end colostomy surgery?" or "What effect does a pain level of 3/10 have on ambulation within four hours of surgery?" Early outcome efforts ought to focus on populations that are high cost and high volume, because this target population is likely to demonstrate the most profound results. Once a measurable outcome has been identified, one can proceed to outcome measurement activities.

Outcome measurement can be the most difficult step in this process. It is important to the success of the project not to allow this to become a stumbling block to progress. A variety of different tools can be used to measure the nature of the problem identified. Instruments may include tools for recording demographics, laboratory values, functional status of the patient, variances, patient or family satisfaction, or treatment and procedure protocols. Measurement needs to occur before and after the management effort as this will provide the clinician with cost, clinical, or satisfaction data through which to demonstrate value of the change to be introduced.

Outcome management is the most exciting part of the outcome effort. It is the point in which clinicians are able to introduce a change that is thought to improve the quality of patient care, based on the pilot measurement. This is why it is so important in outcome identification, the first step of this process, to identify a problem that is measurable. For example, consider the question posed earlier: "What percent of patients with a BMI of 45 to 55, having surgery longer than three hours develop skin injury within the first three postoperative days?" Let's assume that the clinician discovered that 40 percent of the defined patient popula-

tion developed skin injury, costing the facility an average of $10,000 for each patient. Now let's assume that the clinician introduced a change that decreased the incidence of skin injury among the defined population by 75 percent, resulting in a considerable cost savings to the facility. In addition to the cost benefit, important secondary benefits can occur. For example, the clinician may use this information to justify not only his or her position within the facility, but to show an improvement in the quality of care provided to this patient population.

### GETTING STARTED

Assuming the clinician is interested in pursuing outcome efforts, how does one get started? The best way to approach this is to assemble a team of individuals who are interested in the same effort. Experts from a variety of disciplines can be helpful in creating a diverse team. Individuals closest to the process need to be involved because they can better relate the real life concerns that occur. For example, if the team is considering mobility challenges among bariatric patients, membership could include someone from a lift team, a nurses aid who is responsible for mobilizing the patient, or a physi-

cal therapist who understands the physiology of mobilizing the bariatric patient. Each of these individuals is able to provide the team with front-line input.

Outcome identification is an important step for reasons described previously, and the value of the team is that members can define the problem with the greatest clarity because of their various backgrounds. The same with outcome measurement and management. A team is considered a valuable resource to these efforts.

### OPPORTUNITIES

A variety of opportunities are available that will assist the clinician in caring for the bariatric patient. For reasons described earlier, the bariatric patient poses a number of common and predictable complications in healthcare settings. For example, wouldn't it be interesting to find out what percentage of morbidly obese patients actually develop complications? One might measure the prevalence of patients with a BMI greater than 40. Once the prevalence is determined, the clinician could measure the incidence of skin injury among patients with a BMI of 40 to 50, 51 to 60, 61 to 70, and 70 or above. The question this raises is "What is the incidence of skin injury among hospitalized patients with a BMI of 40 to 50?" and so on. In this case, the clinician can establish the point in which patients begin to develop complications. Intuition tells us that skin injury probably occurs with greater frequency among patients with a greater BMI, but this should be substantiated through outcome measurement. Or perhaps, instead of strictly looking at BMI as a criterion, maybe use of a functional index is more revealing. In other words, limited functional ability may be a more accurate predictor of skin injury. One might discover that a patient can have a very high BMI, but if they are able to turn, transfer, and ambulate, the incidence of skin injury is low. Therefore, if the clinician was introducing a criteria-based protocol for use of bariatric equipment, he or she might want to use both BMI and functional status as the criteria for selecting appropriate equipment.

Another area of increasing interest is caregiver injury. This is a cost outcome; however, because of the fear of injury, caregivers may be reluctant to turn, transfer, or ambulate patients who are very heavy or unstable. This reluctance could lead to immobility-related injury. The question that was raised ear-

lier and applies here is, "What effect does introduction of a lift/transfer system have on caregiver injury when caring for a patient with a BMI greater than 45?" or "What role does a lift resource team have on caregiver injury when caring for a patient with a BMI greater than 45?" All of these are important questions, but without outcome measurement, it is difficult to manage the actual problems.

Consider patient outcomes in measuring the effectiveness and appropriateness of pain assessment and management. Ask clinical units to include pain in their quality improvement plans. Establish policies and procedures that support the appropriate prescription of pain medications. The pain care committee is responsible for ensuring that physicians prescribe appropriate analgesics. The committee reviews and revises policies and procedures to assure that all patients receive the best possible pain relief within the realm of safety. This approach is coupled with education of physicians about alternatives to risky and ineffective methods of managing pain. A policy that restricts meperidine use often is reviewed. Revising intravenous patient-controlled analgesia order forms is often a helpful way to

guide physicians in the prescription of appropriate drugs and dosages. A pain care committee is one mechanism for promoting an interdisciplinary approach to improving pain management throughout an institution.

## CHALLENGES TO CLINICIANS

Clinicians are faced with a number of challenges in outcome activities, especially when considering the bariatric patient.[9] The lack of evidence-based practice around caring for the bariatric patient can be problematic in that there is little to no research to support many of our activities. For example, are the mechanisms for wound healing different in the very large patient? What are the ideal interface pressures for the bariatric patient when considering pressure reduction surfaces? Does the use of oversized equipment result in decreased time to mobility or decreased length of stay? Are coping mechanisms the same among the obese and nonobese patient? Unfortunately, there are more questions than answers; however, these questions really offer opportunities for outcome activities.

## THE POWER OF CHANGE

In order to improve the healthcare provided to the

bariatric patient, clinicians must begin to investigate the relationship between what care is provided for the patient and what the measurable outcome is. This is the value of outcome activities.

Payers, providers, and patients are increasingly interested in the study of health outcomes. From the payer's perspective, outcome-based healthcare allows for prediction of resource consumption among patient populations. It sets a standard for clinicians to strive for.

Outcome activities will effect social expectations for greater patient empowerment and public policy. Reimbursement and other important public policy changes are not likely without substantial evidence through outcome efforts.

## CONCLUSION

In conclusion, the clinician best serves the bariatric patient when outcome activities are pursued. Communication of these activities is crucial. This communication can occur in the form of oral or poster presentations, publications, or verbal communications. As we look to improve the quality of care for the bariatric patient, it will be increasingly evident that there is a lack of evidenced-based practice. Outcome research will be necessary to build this pool of necessary evidence. Cost sensitive care that addresses clinical and satisfaction outcomes will continue to be an important element in patient care, and especially bariatric patient care as a high-volume, high-cost population.

## REFERENCES

1. McPheeter M, Lohr KN. Evidence-based Practice and Nursing: Commentary. *Outcomes Management for Nursing Practice* 1999;3:99–101.
2. Nies, MA, Cook T, Bach CA, et al. Concept analysis for advanced practice nursing. *Outcomes Management for Nursing Practice* 1999;3:83–6.
3. Mark BA. The black box of patient outcomes research. Image: *J Nurs Scholarship* 1995;27:42.
4. Campbell ML. Program assessment through outcomes analysis: Efficacy of a comprehensive supportive care team for end-of-life care. *AACN Clinical Issues* 1996;7:159–67.
5. Sousa KH. Description of a health-related quality of life conceptual model. *Outcomes Management for Nursing Practice* 1999;3:78–82.
6. Harris MD. Clinical and financial outcomes in-patient care in a home health agency. *J Nurs Qual Assur* 1991;5:41–9.
7. Wojner AW. Outcomes management: An interdisciplinary search for best practice. *AACN Clinical Issues* 1996;7:133–45.
8. Gallagher SM. Surviving redesign: Basic concepts of patient-focused care and their application to WOC nursing. *JWOCN* 1997;24:132–6.
9. Gallagher SM. Tailoring care for obese patients. *RN* 1999;62:43-45.
10. Effective dashboards can drive improved hospital performance. Available at: www.hfma.org/publications/HFMA_WantsYouToKnow/020905.htm. Access date: June 2005.

# 15

# Ethics

Ethics, by definition, is the philosophic study of morality. It is the study of goodness, moral values, and right action. Morality, on the other hand, arises from the sense of right and wrong actions and good and bad character; therefore, it is concerned with the judgment of the rightness or wrongness of human action and the rightness or wrongness of human character. Morals are usually described as rules or habits of conduct, in regard to right or wrong. Moral principles govern our choices. Moral dilem-

mas arise when a group or an individual has to decide between two or more equally unacceptable choices. Consider the 42-year-old, 520-pound woman who can no longer live at home because severe osteoarthritis interferes with her ability to walk, stand, or perform a reasonable level of activity, including meal preparation and toileting. Leaving her to care for herself is not a good choice, and neither is placing an alert 42-year-old woman in an assisted living facility. A choice between two equally unac-

## UNDERSTANDING OTHERNESS—PETER'S STORY

"My name is Peter, and I have been obese all of my life. I know the meaning of being very different. The way people feel about me is no secret. I see it in their faces. Although children's reactions are the worst, the responses from healthcare professionals can be very painful. Sadly, when I need empathy and compassion the most, I usually don't get it because of my physical appearance. I tend to avoid seeking healthcare because of these reactions. Some professionals will express their feelings about my weight verbally; others will just stare, or worse they will make an effort to peer around the corner to get a good look at me. Other people act as if I am invisible. This distancing is noticeable even among those who are trying to be kind; they will take care not to touch me or make eye contact with me. It is as though my obesity is contagious even to those who try to reach out to me. I find it difficult to accept recommendations for healthcare from a professional who finds me so repulsive. I feel abandoned by those I need the most, which is very disappointing and unfortunate."

Peter holds feelings typical of those who stand outside of the dominant culture—those whose lives possess the quality of otherness. Otherness holds special meaning in healthcare. When clinicians designate the quality of otherness to a patient or patient group, clinicians justify inadequate care and emotional involvement by blaming the patient for the numerous management challenges the patient presents. Like Peter, patients suffering from drug addiction, AIDS, obesity, lung cancer, and other chronic conditions may be excluded or abandoned, particularly in terms of protocols, reimbursement, care, and support because these are often considered self-inflicted conditions.

For more reading on issues of abandonment, exclusion, and otherness, please see:
1. Fanon F. *The Wretched of the Earth.* Harmondsworth, England: Penguin, 1967.
2. Gallagher S. The meaning of otherness in healthcare planning. *Ostomy Wound Manage* 1999;45:18–20.
3. Taylor C. *Multiculturalism.* Princeton, NJ: Princeton University Press, 1994.
4. Volf M. *Exclusion and Embrace: A Theological Exploration of Identity.* Nashville, TN: Abington Press, 1996.

in real choices have to be made with or for real people.

Before the widespread introduction of advanced scientific technology, it was sufficient for intuition and common sense to guide decisions pertaining to dilemmas of right and wrong.[1] Technological advances in healthcare, widespread pluralism, and increasing legal pressure to meet an acceptable standard of care have paved the way for a more systematic approach to ethical decision making.[2,3] Today's proliferation of ethical training and debate, ethics committees and consultation, and other conflict resolution and guidance mechanisms highlight important considerations for what these mechanisms should and should not do, how they should operate, and how they can most successfully function in an evolving practice setting.[4]

The Georgetown Mantra serves as a model to frame ethical dilemmas associated with healthcare decision making and thus can be applied in making decisions in caring for the obese patient. Beneficence, nonmaleficence, respect for personal autonomy, and justice comprise the Georgetown Mantra. Beneficence is the ethical principle that refers to doing good for the patient—the obligation to do those activi-

ceptable choices must be made, and that choice is likely to be made using ethical principles, such as paternalism, respect for personal autonomy, and beneficence. This case represents an example of applied clinical ethics, where-

ties that promote good for the patient. Nonmaleficence refers to the moral obligation to do no harm—not simply to do good, but to protect from harm. Some contend that this means physical harm, but in the care of obese patients, clinicians have an obligation to protect the patient from emotional harm as well. Respect for personal autonomy is an important ethical ideal, particularly among Americans. The US Constitution is grounded on principles of respect for personal autonomy, and thus ideals of autonomy have become an integral part of American culture. Justice in the healthcare setting refers to the just or fair distribution of healthcare goods and services. Principles of justice help stakeholders decide who gets what.

This chapter presents debate pertaining to topics, such as unproven/experimental treatment, access to treatment/care, reasonable accommodation, just/fair distribution of healthcare goods and services, difference, and mutually responsive decision making.

## ABOVE ALL DO NO HARM

Beneficence is described as acts of mercy, kindness, or charity. It is the moral obligation to act for the benefit of others.[5] Benevolence, by con-

trast, is a personal quality described as being there for others or to act for the benefit of others. While the acts of beneficence are not obligatory, the principle of beneficence mandates an obligation to help patients advance their unique personal and legitimate healthcare goals. Obligations of nonmaleficence are considered to be more stringent than obligations of beneficence—typically overriding—but the weights of these moral principles, like all moral principles, vary in different circumstances. Obligations not to harm others are clearly distinct from obligations to help others. In real world healthcare settings, things are not as distinct. Balancing benefit and burden can be complicated when the clinical outcome is uncertain. Consider Dillon Baxter, a 74-year-old, 320-pound man with funds available to privately pay for his requests for bariatric weight loss surgery. For the past three months, he has experienced sleep apnea, lower leg swelling with cellulitis, and fatigue. Prior to that time, however, Dillon had been active, playing golf four times a week, playing handball daily with his grandson, and performing other activities that required physical and mental stamina. He has been to four cities and interviewed 11

bariatric surgeons. He reports that he understands the risks of BWLS at the age of 74, but since his recent change in health status, each physician felt the risks were unacceptably high despite the patient's request.

*Prinum non nocere*, sometimes interpreted to mean "above all, do no harm," is a maxim frequently used by clinicians. The maxim "Do no harm" describes the ethical principle of nonmaleficence. As options in healthcare continue to incorporate advances in medical technology, discussions about the benefit/burden balance become increasingly more important, especially in terms of the obligation to do no harm. Differences in the perception of health and healthcare differ from one person to another because of religion, educational, cultural, and experiential differences, or in Mr. Baxter's situation, difference in economic status.

At issue is what constitutes nonmaleficence and beneficence in the presence of chronic conditions, such as obesity, because some treatments may hold unproven benefits, such as surgical intervention among older obese patients. Little or no evidence exists to describe the outcomes of BWLS among 74-year-old morbidly obese patients with a recent decline in health. Like all ethical dilemmas, there is no acceptable choice in Mr Baxter's case.

## JUST DISTRIBUTION OF HEALTHCARE GOODS AND SERVICES

Justice is described as fairness, and distributive justice refers to the just distribution of healthcare goods and services, especially in the face of scarce resources. In caring for the bariatric patient, this refers to the just distribution of goods and services as it pertains to the care of larger, heavier patients, regardless of practice setting. It is about the specially designed outpatient room that accommodates the larger patient with wounds related to lipolymphedema, or the oversized operating room table for the 600-pound patient with appendicitis, or the 94-inch abdominal binder for the new mother in the post-partum unit. Problems of distributive justice arise under conditions of scarcity or competition. The goal is to balance burden (cost and the needs of other protected groups) with benefit, which is likely to be a clinical outcome. A trade-off or compromise is inevitable. For example, consider the hospital that eliminates the bariatric coordinator position with thoughts of sharing

those responsibilities between the lab, admitting, and the house supervisor. Those patients and clinicians closest to the service line understand the consequence. From an ethical perspective, how can cost of a service be balanced with the clinical outcome of the service? In light of limited or scarce resources, how can a fair compromise be made? Questions about who should receive what share of the nation's scarce resources continues to spark debate about a national health plan, unequal distribution of advantages to the disadvantaged, and the rationing of healthcare. Debate is generated about access and distribution of health insurance and health insurance coverage, and costs of specialized treatment, such as BWLS or Wellness Centers.

Some contend that the reason many obese people have little access to valuable healthcare goods and services is because they speak in a voice that is not heard. Insurance carriers have recently made efforts to reduce access to BWLS for a number of debatable reasons. From an ethical perspective, it becomes the obligation of clinicians to speak in a voice that is heard by those limiting accessing in a language that is understood. Additionally,

consumers are learning to do the same. Groups such as the Council for Size and Weight Discrimination (www.cswd.org) and others are providing a unified voice to those who are responsible for making decisions about allocation of scarce resources. Inequalities in access to healthcare and health insurance, combined with the dramatic increases in the cost of healthcare, fueled debates about social justice in the US and other countries. Clinicians are important stakeholders in this debate and they are likely to speak for the patient who has been literally or politically silenced.

## UNPROVEN TREATMENT

The value of evidence-based practice is the extent to which clinicians and patients are confident that the selected treatment or procedure is likely to have merit in meeting the patient's needs. However, the dilemma among many obese patients is that some will seek any available treatment, regardless of safety or evidence of therapeutic value. This poses dilemmas of an ethical nature in that clinicians have an obligation to protect patients from harm-nonmaleficence, but the concept of futility also should be considered.

Consider Sara, a 27-year-old elementary school teacher with a BMI of 52. She reports that not only do the children make fun of her, but so do their parents. She recently reported that she has lost thousands of pounds throughout her life, but becomes uncomfortable with unwelcome attention when she begins to lose weight. Sara is asking for a referral to a bariatric weight loss surgery center in hopes that surgery will resolve her weight issues. You explain that surgery is just a tool, and that weight loss following BWLS requires a tremendous amount of effort. You believe she would benefit from psychological counseling before BWLS. She further explains that she has met someone who is interested in her, but he is hesitant to become more involved with her because of her weight. In the event that Sara began psychological therapy, resolved her emotional issues, and then went on to have BWLS, no ethical decision or debate would be necessary; however, clinicians know this seldom happens. Sara's situation, as it is presented, holds numerous opportunities for ethical debate, and as with every ethical dilemma, a decision must be made from several equally unacceptable choices. Certainly one could remind readers that the decision is

ultimately Sara's and would appeal to respect for personal autonomy. If Sara wants a referral for BWLS, she should have that granted; on the other hand, what about non-maleficence, or the duty to protect patients from harm? Patients like Sara who weight cycle because of underlying emotional issues with thinness struggle with BWLS because the underlying factors prevent the patient from feeling comfortable with their new, thinner appearance.

Some patients claim entitlement to any care they desire, regardless of success or outcome. Some clinicians refuse to prescribe certain treatments because the treatment is thought to be futile. Prescribing or offering futile therapy breaks trust with patients and families, exploits fear, inflates the realistic boundaries of what intervention can be accomplished, enhances the illusion of patient autonomy, and interferes with the clinician's ability to meaningfully help the patient.[6] The central theme of healthcare is to help patients and their families. Therefore, beneficence is critical to the concept of healthcare. Those who prescribe treatment that they recognize will not improve the patient's condition break trust with the patient and undercut the very meaning of care. If the

patient is misled to believe in a treatment's efficacy, the patient's trust is breached.

Recent debate pertaining to futility has been useful in clarifying the clinician's responsibility to communicate, educate, establish trust, and collaborate with the goal of mutually responsive decision making.[7] As care and treatment for obese individuals becomes more complex and readily available, it becomes increasingly important for clinicians to understand indications for treatment tools and the way they correspond with the unique needs of the patient. Clinicians are in a key position to identify issues of futility and can often avoid unnecessary conflict through open, honest communication. In cases where reasonable resolution cannot be reached through meaningful communication and trust, institutions appeal to ethics committees or case conferences to provide guidance to clinicians, patients, and their families.

## ROLE OF THE ETHICS COMMITTEE

From a historical perspective, ethics committees are not a recent phenomenon; however, some believe they gained increasing popularity in 1976, shortly after the decision of *In the Matter of*

*Karen Quinlan*,[8] which launched an era of open discussion about legal and ethical issues that arise out of healthcare delivery. Karen Ann Quinlan was a 21-year-old woman who had a cardiopulmonary arrest in 1975 and died 10 years later, never regaining consciousness. Her parents sought permission from the courts to allow her to die naturally by removing ventilatory support. The Quinlans won their case, and the ventilatory support was removed. Ms. Quinlan died nine years later. This case dramatized the moral and legal debate over life-sustaining treatment after the irreversible loss of all meaningful cognitive functions.

At the time of the Quinlan case, it was recommended that hospitals form ethics committees as a means to serve and advise providers. This was supported by the President's Committee for the Study of Ethical Problems in Medicine and Biomedical and Behavioral Research.[9] In addition, accreditation standards of the Joint Commission on Accreditation of Healthcare Organizations and legislation in some states require hospitals to have a mechanism for conflict resolution and guidance on ethical issues.

The main role of an ethics committee consultation is to promote communication among patients, families, and clinicians regarding treatment decisions and to assist in the decision-making process when ethical conflicts arise. An ethics committee consultation is strictly advisory and is intended to assist in the decision-making process by examining facts, while balancing the ethical principles and personal beliefs within the context of the strong emotions often involved in the situation. A consultation can also be requested when the patient's views about his or her long-term care options conflict with the views of family members, or when a clinician and a patient or family member have differing opinions regarding medical treatment.

Ethics committees are generally interdisciplinary in nature and likely comprise physicians, nurses, administrators, social workers, psychologists, respiratory therapists, clergy, trustees, attorneys, ethicist, patient advocates, and community members. These committees should combine the expertise and perspectives of a number of different individuals from a variety of different disciplines. When addressing concerns of a bariatric patient, an unbiased clinician with an expertise in care for obese patients would serve an ethics committee well.

Patients and clinicians have the right to expect that all communication, whether written or verbal, which pertains to the situation will be held in strictest confidence. In some hospitals, confidentiality is a factor in determining the place of the ethics committee within the institution's organizational structure. For example, if records of administration or governance committees are subject to public disclosure, then establishing an ethics committee as a medical staff committee with a multidisciplinary membership would more likely ensure confidentiality.[10]

Anna is a 400-pound 47-year-old woman who was admitted to acute care through the emergency department with stage IV necrotic pressure ulcers to the buttocks and stage III open pressure ulcers with slough to the hips, in the perineal folds, and the mid-back. Additionally, she has developed cellulitis to the abdomen, right neck, and lower legs. Living at home by herself, she was unable to care for her skin, prepare meals, and engage in other basic activities of daily living. In the intensive care unit, she was provided with hygienic care, antibiotics, hydration, parenteral nutrition, and ventilation. Her condition continued to deteriorate with a pulse rate of 140, blood pressure 70/40, and cool, pale skin. The dilemma in question is local wound care to the necrotic buttocks. The standard of care for necrotic-covered pressure ulcers dictates removal of necrotic material with subsequent reduction of bacterial load.[11] However, debridement would entail aggressive local treatment. Once the wound was unroofed, there would be considerable drainage and odor. Without debridement, bacteria can multiply rapidly in the presence of such a profound amount of necrotic matter. Therein lies the dilemma. The current national standard does not best serve the patient's needs. Clinicians talked with Sara's family to explain the dilemma Sara's condition posed both legal and moral dilemmas. Her family seemed satisfied with the plan of care, which included continued critical care intervention including antibiotics for the widespread cellulitis, pressure relief, nutrition, hydration, and personal hygiene. Aggressive local wound care to the buttocks would be deferred to that time when Sara's overall physical condition might improve.

The wound care clinician and physician wondered what legal and ethical implications arose out of this situation.

Each was reminded that legal and risk management issues must be addressed separately from moral issues. Legal counsel was consulted, but additionally both agreed to present their concerns to the hospital ethics committee. The function of an ethics committee is to assist clinicians facing a variety of dilemmas. In this case, the committee served as a resource for the two clinicians. It was apparent that the principal stakeholders involved in the dilemma were satisfied with the plan of care; however, the wound care clinician was not confident that everyone understood that wounds like Sara's are likely to open and exude highly odorous drainage. This can create undue stress on caregivers, visitors, and the patient.

The ethics committee broached this dilemma using models readily available for encouraging ethical discussion and debate. The ethics committee achieved the following three goals in this case: 1) clarified the ethical issue(s), 2) contributed to improved patient care, and 3) mentored in decision-making skills.

Through discussion, the wound care clinician expressed he wasn't uncomfortable with the plan of care so much as the potential mis-

understanding Sara's family might have regarding the gravity of this skin complication. The clinician explained he had concerns pertaining to the ethical principle of informed consent. Did the family, and even other clinicians, really understand the physiologic impact of a wound of this magnitude? The committee offered the necessary support the clinician needed. The ethics committee suggested to the wound care clinician that he might make himself available to clinicians and the family as needed. The ultimate plan of patient care was to best serve Sara's needs and to recognize the difficulty uncertainty poses in decision making. This entailed adding the option for wound care consultation to the existing plan of care.

Most would agree that the Committee should not substitute for decisions made at the patient/clinician level. Ideally, clinicians will learn from experiences with ethics committees and develop their own ability to clarify ethical issues, discuss them together with their patients, and continue to provide the highest level of patient care—care that truly reflects the needs of the patient.

## SUMMARY
The challenge of dealing

with ethics within the healthcare setting and within society continues in complexity. Clinicians are faced with ethical dilemmas with increasing frequency. As advanced technology moves into this arena of specialized care, this will grow increasingly apparent. Clinicians may consider resources to assist in making decisions, such as ethics committees. Ethics committees, on the other hand, may seek the expertise of bariatric clinicians, in hopes of better understanding the complexities in caring for larger, heavier patients and the implications of caring for the patient experiencing the many issues associated with obesity.

Communication, whether with the patient, significant other, peers, ethics consultants, committees or some other form of conflict resolution, can lead to a more successful patient/clinician relationship. Ethical principles, education, professional debate, ethics committees, and consultation are resources that encourage this ethical responsiveness.

## REFERENCES

1.  Jonsen AR, Siegler M, Winslade WJ. *Clinical Ethics, Second Edition.* New York, NY: Macmillan Publishing Company, 1985.
2.  La Puma J, Scheidermayer DL, Toulmin SE, et al. The standard of care: A case report and ethical analysis. *Ann Intern Med* 1988;108:121–4.
3.  Purtillo RB. Ethics consultation in the hospital. *N Eng J Med* 1984;311:983–6.
4.  American Hospital Association. *Values in Conflict: Resolving Ethical issues in Health Care, 2nd ed.* (AHA Catalog No. C - 0250002).Chicago, IL: American Hospital Publishing, 1993.
5.  Beachamp TL & Childress JF. *Principles of Biomedical Ethics.* New York: NY: Oxford University Press, 2000:260.
6.  Schneiderman LJ, Jecker NS, Jonson AR. Medical futility: Its meaning and ethical implications. *Ann Int Med* 1990;112:949–54.
7.  Coppa S. Futile care. *JONA* 1996;26:18–23.
8.  In re: Quinlan, 70 NJ 10, 355 A2d 647(1976) cert denied, 429 US 922 (1976).
9.  President's Commission for the Study of Ethical Problems in Medicine and Biomedical Research: Deciding to Forego Life-Sustaining Treatment: *Ethical, Medical, and Legal Issues in Treatment Decisions* 1983;440–56.
10. American Hospital Association. *Values in Conflict: Resolving Ethical issues in Health Care, 2nd ed.* (AHA Catalog No. C - 0250002).Chicago:American Hospital Publishing;1993.
11. US Agency for Health Care Policy and Research. *Treating Pressure Sores. Clinical Practice Guideline* (AHCPR No. 95-0654). Rockville, MD, Department of Health and Human Services, 1994.

# 16

# Legal Realities

**E**xperts from *Lawyers Weekly USA* explain, "Medical malpractice claims over obesity surgery are on the rise as more and more severely obese patients turn to weight loss surgery for rapid weight loss." For instance, the family of a Lancaster, New Hampshire, man who died seven days after BWLS reportedly won a $900,000 verdict against a hospital that failed to give him medication he had been taking prior to surgery. However, jury results have been mixed in awards. In a recent defense victory, an Orleans Parish, Louisiana, jury found that the death of an obese patient four days after BWLS was caused by problems unrelated to the surgery itself. Some attorneys are wary of representing plaintiffs in negligence cases involving obese patients. Regardless, clinicians must begin to acknowledge and address efforts to ensure legally sound practice. This chapter reviews the legal theory of negligence, including the four elements of a claim. Documentation, communication, informed consent and

## UNDERSTANDING RISKS

Some of the most common reasons for claims include 1) deep vein thrombosis (DVT) or other embolic condition, which result in death, 2) pressure ulcer development, and 3) failure to recognize anastomic leak, which results in sepsis. Certainly patients file claims for many reasons; however, claims of negligence pertaining to care of the bariatric patient often fall into one of these three categories. Some experts believe that DVT is more prevalent among the morbidly obese, so the plaintiff's attorney will call those experts to testify. Therefore, what is important to clinicians is that DVT prophylaxis must be addressed, communicated, and documented. If the physician has ordered ambulation, it is no longer appropriate to document, "Patient too large to ambulate." Resources to begin the mobility process, regardless of the patient's weight, do exist.

Clinicians must recognize that patients will develop pressure ulcers if they are unable to turn, because of the pain they are in, they are uncooperative, or they are obtunded. Additionally, otherwise healthy patients who are placed in hospital beds that are too narrow are unable to reposition themselves. These patients are also likely to develop pressure ulcers, especially in the buttock cleft. These often go undetected until after the patient is discharged home. What a surprise at the first post-operative office visit! If the patient could turn, but can't because of the width of the bed, consider a wider frame with a simple foam surface.

The overwhelming nature of complex patients makes it important to pay close attention to every system and to use a formula to approach assessment. Infection or anastomotic leak must be suspect any time the patient develops hypotension, tachycardia, increased respirations, and elevated body temperature. In the event this sequelae develops, the surgeon must be notified in an urgent manner.

Although there is never absolute protection against litigation, documentation that the standards of care were met, regardless of the patient's size or weight, offers a reasonable defense.

## DOCUMENTATION

Attorneys and other experts look to the chart to determine the story of a patient's healthcare experience, whether it's in the hospital, clinic, or home. Timely, accurate, and legible documentation is imperative. It is always a disappointment to the defense when documentation to turning and repositioning occurred for the five-hour period after the patient had expired. Remember the mantra, "Do what you say, say what you do!" In the event there are questions as to what to document or how to document a special event, it may be in your best interest to speak with your risk manager. This is especially true in situations where there are issues of adherence.

informed refusal are discussed. Case studies and resources are included.

Historically, larger Americans have been reluctant to bring attention to themselves. From a legal perspective, many obese patients feel they are responsible for inadequate care because of their weight. However, in the past few years, size and weight acceptance advocates are asserting the legal right to equal accommodation, demanding the same standards of care regardless of body size or weight. The legal system provides a means for larger Americans to test this claim, and many times the claim is against the healthcare community. Satisfied, informed consumers are less likely to file a claim against healthcare institutions or clinicians, and therefore the failure to communicate is often at the heart of litigation as is inadequate documentation.

## UNDERSTANDING NEGLIGENCE

Negligence is the most common legal theory used in medical malpractice cases. This theory can be applied not only in medical malpractice cases, but personal injury cases, and defendants in these cases could be individuals, organizations, or manufacturers. Usually, many defendants are named. In order to win a negligence suit, the plaintiff's attorney must prove that four legal elements exist.

## LEGAL ELEMENTS OF A CLAIM

Even before a claim is filed, an attorney will screen the case for suitability. Four elements must be present in order for the attorney to consider the merits of the case, which are duty, breach of duty, damages, and causation. In order to ensure the duty element is satisfied, a relationship must exist between the clinician (defendant) and the patient/family member (plaintiff). The clinician holds a duty to perform consistently with an established standard of care (SOC).

A breach of duty exists when there has been a negligent departure from a recognized SOC. A breach of duty might also then be defined as the failure to do what the reasonable and prudent person possessing the same or similar skills and knowledge would do in the same or similar circumstances.

If the attorney determines that a breach of duty has occurred, then he or she will determine if damages have actually occurred and to what extent. The purpose of granting damages is to compensate and provide restitution for

**BOOK REVIEW**

Beckman JP. *Nursing negligence: Analyzing malpractice in the hospital setting.* Thousand Oaks, CA: Sage Publications,1996.

Beckman describes the origins of nursing malpractice and the morbidity and mortality associated with it. *Nursing Negligence* takes a no-nonsense approach to the legal aspects of malpractice and presents an overview of common nursing malpractice issues. The author appeals to nurses to accept nursing standards and to address the very real problems of negligence. She defines nursing malpractice and demonstrates how it can be identified and prevented across practice settings. Using both quantitative and qualitative methods, the author presents research findings from actual malpractice cases in a clear and approachable manner. Beckman addresses common adverse nursing care outcomes, characteristics of patients with negative outcomes, cost associated with malpractice litigation, departures from standard care that cause injury and death, and risk prevention strategies.

Leaman TL, Saxton JW. *Preventing Malpractice: The CO-Active Solution.* Norwell, MA: Kluwer Academic Publishers, 2001.

Written by a family practice physician and an attorney, this book serves as a practical guide to primary care physicians on how to how to weave time-effective and cost-efficient risk management principles into daily practice. Despite the intended audience, the authors offer ideas that are useful for nurses, risk managers, and others. Advice is offered to prevent lawsuits, recognize risks, and prepare for deposition and trial. The valuable underlying theme is a risk management strategy that emphasizes a partnership role between physicians and their patients, which stresses communication and documentation.

**WHAT IS A STANDARD OF CARE (SOC)?**

When locating a standard of care, attorneys and their experts look to standards that have been adopted by legislation, case law, professional organizations, institutional policies and procedures, and national standards of care. By definition, a standard of care is that standard which holds a person of exceptional skill or knowledge to a duty of acting as would a reasonable and prudent person possessing the same or similar skills or knowledge under the same or similar circumstances. For purposes of this lengthy legal definition, a "reasonable and prudent person" is thought to be a person who exercises skill with reasonable care, diligence, and judgment. However, a standard of care is not the clinician's own personal judgment, and it is not based on a local or community standard; it is a national standard. Therefore, a community or local standard is not a legal standard. This is especially true now due to the widespread use of the Internet, which creates a national community.

## INFORMED CONSENT

Patients and their families are becoming increasingly responsible partners in healthcare. Communication about options for managing obesity and understanding its nature is more important than ever. State laws have been developed to govern communication between clinicians, patients, and their family members/friends. Commonly referred to as informed consent laws, these laws specify the types of information that patients must be provided so that patients can make informed decisions about care, diagnostic studies, or treatment. Informed consent is the process by which fully informed patients can participate in choices about their healthcare. It originates from the legal and ethical right the patient has in directing what happens to her body and from the ethical duty of the clinician to involve the patient in her care. The most important goal of informed consent is that patients have an opportunity to be informed participants in their care decisions. It is generally accepted that complete informed consent includes a discussion of the following elements:

- The nature of the decision/procedure
- Reasonable alternatives to the proposed intervention
- Relative risk benefits and uncertainties of each alternative
- Assessment of patient understanding
- Acceptance of the intervention by the patient.

In order for the patient's consent to be valid, she must be considered competent to make the decision and the consent must be voluntary. It is easy for coercive situations to arise in medicine. Patients often feel powerless and vulnerable; therefore, to encourage voluntariness, the clinician can make clear to the patient that she is participating in a decision, not merely signing a form. With this understanding, clinicians must take care to ensure the patient has been given adequate information, both written and verbal, and has sufficient opportunity to ask questions and clarify information.

For more on informed consent:
www.medicalmalpractice.net/sections/resources/informedconsent.htm

wrongdoing. In some cases, damages are granted to punish wrongdoers and deter further wrongdoing. Plaintiffs in a negligence case are entitled to recover any damages that can be proven. This would include economic, noneconomic, or punitive damages.

Economic damages are usually pretty straightforward and may include medical expenses, lost wages, rehabilitation costs, or funeral expenses. It could be more difficult to place a monetary amount on noneconomic damages, such as pain and suffering, lost

love or companionship, and hedonic damages. Hedonic damages are considered lost pleasure and loss of enjoyment. Punitive damages are not always applicable, but when awarded, it is thought to punish the defendant and deter further misconduct.

Despite the fact that the first three elements are present, it is still necessary for the attorney to prove to the jury that causation exists. The plaintiff must prove a direct causal relationship between the acts of negligence and the alleged damages. This is done in two ways. The first is described by the notion of foreseeability; the plaintiff must prove that the defendant should have foreseen that the negligence could result in the alleged damages. The second way causation is proven is by making the following statement: In reasonable probability, the damages would not have occurred but for the negligence. In some parts of the country, this is also stated as the defendant's negligence being a substantial factor in causing the alleged damages.

## ISSUES OF ADHERENCE

Caring for larger patients is certainly more complex. Even without any coexisting diagnoses or preadmission mobility issues, care can be complicated sometimes simply due to a patient's body weight. Patients and caregivers are asked to perform tasks that they may be ill equipped to achieve. This raises questions of adherence. Sometimes the inability to accomplish activities because of patient-related fear or apprehension is labeled nonadherence. It is important to try to differentiate this from a patient's refusal to participate in care. For example, your patient may refuse to ambulate for fear of falling, as compared to your patient who refuses a physical therapy appointment because it coincides with a special television program. Understanding the difference is challenging in itself.

From a legal perspective, issues of adherence are an important factor. Certainly, they pose documentation challenges. Again, in the case of failure to participate in care, you may need to organize a team conference that would include your risk manager or hospital attorney. This is especially true if the nonadherent behavior influences the clinical outcome. Perhaps as a team, you will discover that the seeming nonadherence is fear of the respective activity. However, if care concerns are not resolved in the team conference, your risk manager

## COMMUNICATION

**B**everly had been heavy her entire life and was thrilled to learn she had been approved to have BWLS. On the day she met the surgeon, she was elated. She never heard him explain that she would need to walk the evening of surgery, she never heard him say she could experience some postoperative pain, and she never heard him explain that she would be off work 4 to 6 weeks, although she signed acknowledgment of the conversation. Her sister Beatrice had the same surgery, or so she thought, and was back at work in seven days. Beatrice actually went home within 24 hours of the Lap-Band procedure. Beverly's surgery went fine for a RNYGB; she had pain levels of three to four most of the four-day hospitalization, and she was back to work in five weeks. Imagine the team's surprise when they discovered Beverly had filed a claim. Suits can be filed for a number of reasons. Some authors contend that misunderstanding is sometimes at the heart of claims. The patient held an expectation that was not met by the healthcare institution or the clinician(s); an adverse outcome that was unexpected occurred. However, the occurrence of an adverse outcome does not prove negligence. Negligence must be proven using the four legal elements. Beverly's claim that the pain was unreasonable and she did not return to work in a reasonable period of time had no merit based on the fact that the four elements were not met. Experts could not identify a breach in the standard of care. Regardless, the claim was disturbing from a number of perspectives. Defending against a lawsuit can be costly economically and emotionally. Clinicians are encouraged to offer and document realistic expectations and clarify the patient's understanding, such as to recognize miscommunications.

## AVOIDING RED FLAGS

**M**r. Adams was admitted to the critical care area with a full-thickness pressure ulcer. Staff members were especially concerned because of the difficulty they encountered when repositioning him, as he was 520 pounds and heavily sedated. Rather than coordinating a team conference to orchestrate a team effort, each clinician made recommendations based on their clinical experience with patients similar to Mr. Adams. Within a 24-hour period, the following orders were written on the order sheet: "Please reposition at least every two hours," "Duoderm to buttocks area, change every three days;" "Cleanse with normal saline, dry, and apply enzymatic debriding agent every eight hours;" "Local pulsation therapy to sacral area daily, wet-to-moist dressings." Each of these treatments could be appropriate; however, not all of them at the same time. This type of documentation suggests miscommunication or failure to communicate.  If the medical record suggests there is lack of communication between clinicians, attorneys tend to investigate further. This is considered a "red flag."

## INFORMED REFUSAL

In the face of intervention that holds special risks, it is important to discuss options with the patient and document the discussion to that extent. A patient may choose not to have a particular condition treated. Even if not treating the disease or condition means that the individual will die, US courts have increasingly affirmed the patient's right to reject treatment. Consequently, informed consent laws now include the concept of informed refusal. This means that clinicians must inform the patient of the risks or consequences of refusing treatment or diagnostic tests. It becomes the patient's responsibility to be sure that they understand the information that they have been given, even if it means reviewing the information with the patient several times. A patient-oriented standard disclosure means that the clinician is required to disclose risks, facts, and alternatives that a reasonable person in a reasonable situation would consider important in deciding to have or not to have a recommended treatment.

For more on informed consent, visit The American Cancer Society Website at www.cancer.org.

## MEDICAL MALPRACTICE CLAIMS AND OBESITY SURGERY

Gerner R, Med-mal claims for common obesity surgery of the rise. Accessed at: http://www.slackdavis.com/practice_article.php

can direct the best method to document the situation. This step may protect you and your institution from a lengthy legal encounter.

### SUMMARY

There is no question that clinicians and organizations are continually at risk for legal action; however, there are steps that can be taken to control for non-meritorious claims.

The obese patient holds numerous care challenges, and it is in the interest of healthcare organizations to meet these challenges in a clinically and legally sound manner.

# 17

# Preplanning for Care

**O**bese patients who are hospitalized are reportedly at a higher risk for certain common and predictable complications simply because of their body weight and size.[1] For instance, patients who are 45.4kg (100 pounds) or more above ideal body weight have exponential increases in mortality and serious morbidity as compared with their nonobese counterparts.[2] Because of both emotional and physical issues, some obese people resist pursuing healthcare and frequently defer hospitalization until the last possible moment.[3] Therefore, in many cases, caring for obese patients may be more complicated.

Clinicians recognize that healthcare is fast becoming one of the most dangerous jobs in the US.[4] In acute care facilities, turning, lifting, and repositioning very heavy patients can predispose caregivers to physical injury. This creates a barrier to care in that even the most compassionate caregiver may consider the possibility of caregiver injury when providing care.[5] Despite these concerns, preplanning activities are generally not forthcoming. The value of criteria-based protocols as they are thought to improve care and control costs by preplanning for resource allocation is discussed herein. Barriers to preplanning are addressed. Additionally, strategies for overcoming these barriers are presented, with attention to caregiver injury, interdisciplinary patient care, and associated costs. A criteria-based interdisciplinary protocol is included as well as a first person account that captures the experience of developing a very complex protocol that draws on the expertise of a number of individuals and disciplines.

## BARRIERS TO PREPLANNING

A number of barriers exist to any kind of change in healthcare organizations. The well-documented nursing shortage has posed challenges in all but the most essential performance improvement efforts because clinicians are unable to leave their direct patient care responsibilities to participate in team meetings, data collection, or other activities. The financial instability of many healthcare organizations has further threatened the trend for changes and subsequent improvement in some areas

---

### FIRST PERSON—REAL LIFE CHALLENGES IN DEVELOPING AN INTERDISCIPLINARY PROTOCOL

The challenge in putting together a bariatric criteria-based protocol or preplanning tool is the fact that few clinicians consider themselves bariatric specialists. However, the value of an interdisciplinary team is that every discipline brings a unique and valuable perspective, and together the team becomes expertly prepared to embark on creating a meaningful protocol. In other words, members of the team need to be reminded that even though a specific clinician isn't a bariatric expert, the team is. This is the greatest real life challenge. Once the team recognizes its strength as a team, the work begins. The first assignment was the development of a protocol. The assembled experts developed content sections explicit to their specialty. All drafts were reviewed by the entire team and resulted in a final document that was a seamless process of care between disciplines. The final draft was approved via the appropriate channels.

---

of patient care. Organizations are reluctant to devote resources to services that may not see a positive outcome right away because the immediate bottom line is of the greatest importance. However, one recent study suggests that barriers to preplanning for obese patients may be related to the complex nature of the patient population. It has become difficult to determine how to begin to develop a criteria-based protocol.[6] Consider the departments that ought to be involved; it is likely that every department in the hospital has contact with members of this patient group. For example, whether the patient is admitted through the emergency department or through the admitting office, special accommodation is necessary.

Failure to preplan can hinder patient movement from one department to another, therefore leading to further delays in necessary diagnostic and therapeutic intervention.

## CRITERIA-BASED PROTOCOLS

Getting started can be the most challenging aspect of developing a bariatric protocol. Little to no research exists to describe best practice strategies for care. Clinical experts, teamwork, and group participation are critical to embracing a project of this complexity. Additionally, in striving for success, frontline employees must be part of the process. Change requires strong leadership, active participation, empowerment, and education. Support is essential on

**BARIATRIC INTERDISCIPLINARY ORDER SET**

1.  **Private room**
2.  **WOCN consult within 48 hours**
3.  **Nutrition consult within 24 hours**
4.  **Pharmacy consult within 12 hours**
5.  **Physical therapy/Occupational therapy consult within 24 hours**
6.  **Respiratory therapy consult within 24 hours**
7.  **Case management/social services within 48 hours of admission**
8.  **Interdisciplinary team meeting within 48 hours of admission, and regularly thereafter**
9.  **Equipment within 8 hours of admission**
    **a. Oversized bed to allow space for turning if independent**
       **i. Consider rotation therapy if unable to turn or for pulmonary issues**
       **ii. Consider alternating pressure for skin issues**
    **b. Lift and/or transfer system if unable to exit bed independently**
       **i. Hover-type lateral transfer product**
       **ii. Lift and transfer for complete transfer**
       **iii. Trapeze**
    **c. Walker**
    **d. Wheelchair**
    **e. Commode if in room with wall-mounted toilet or if unable to walk to bathroom**
10. **Notify off-unit diagnostic services two hours before all procedures**
11. **Weigh patient (indicate one) daily QOD weekly**

all levels. Communication between disciplines and departments is imperative.[7] In developing a plan of care, the value of an interdisciplinary team cannot be overlooked. Pharmacists, physical and occupational therapists, podiatrists, and other specialists, including vendors, can offer valuable ideas in preplanning for care. Each discipline brings unique ideas and solutions to common challenges. A team approach has become the standard of care for many organizations. For example, some organizations require interdisciplinary patient care conferences within eight hours of admission if the patient meets certain criteria, such as a body mass index (BMI) greater than 50. However, the presence of a team does not necessarily ensure timely access to assessment and intervention.[8] A preplanning tool becomes the critical factor in caring for more complex patients.

Healthcare facilities should have a plan in place for the special needs of the morbidly obese patient. Patients are best served when resources such as equipment and care are appropriate to the patient's size, weight distribution, and mobility needs. Additionally, consider equipment provided through the organization, such as magnetic resonance imaging (MRI) scanners, operating room tables, or X-ray tables, that typically have weight limitations. Identifying the weight limits of diagnostic and treatment equipment house-wide prevents misunderstandings as to what resources are actually available to clinicians.

Preplanning with manufacturers and vendors to provide equipment for the morbidly obese patient is essential. Institutional policies and procedures for obtaining oversized transportation and transfer devices, bed frames and support surfaces, wheelchairs, walkers, and commodes or furniture need to be instituted.[9] When selecting oversized equipment, it is essential to consider both the weight limits and the width of the equipment. For example, patients not exceeding the weight limit for a standard bedside commode may still be unable to use a standard device due to hip size. Most medical equipment suppliers rent or sell extra-wide wheelchairs, walkers, and commodes that accommodate patients weighing up to 1,000 pounds. Some rental companies provide a number of oversized bariatric items as a bundle, providing a price incentive.

Although appropriate equipment is essential, other resources are equally valuable. Healthcare clinicians and hospital support personnel need to be involved in the preplanning process. Education is critical to planning individualized care that complements the criteria-based protocol. Competency tools can be a resource to set and maintain standards of care.

## MAKING CHANGES

Despite education, clinical skills, and special resources, challenges to delivering safe, effective skin and wound care exist. Clinicians across the country are discovering that solutions to these costly and preventable complications are not forthcoming. Criteria-based protocols, policies, or procedures typically assist in providing a meaningful standard of care for complex costly patient groups by employing a consistent process for delivering care

### ACCESS TO DIAGNOSTIC/PROCEDURAL AREAS

Elizabeth had been transferred from a rural acute care hospital to the rehabilitation unit in a busy urban medical center. At 375 pounds, it was thought that this change better provided necessary resources to facilitate Elizabeth's recovery. On Day 2 of her rehabilitation, a physician order for gym-based physical therapy was generated. The nurses prepared Elizabeth for her first treatment. There was an excitement in the air as a bariatric lift and transfer system was used to effortlessly transfer Elizabeth from the bed to wheelchair; the oversized wheelchair easily and safely transported Elizabeth to the gym. The excitement waned when the physical therapist discovered Elizabeth's weight and girth. Although there were resources in the facility to manage her needs, the department hadn't had the opportunity to preplan for Elizabeth's arrival. If the clinical staff had understood Elizabeth's needs, at the very least the oversized lift could have been available along with additional staff and provisions for privacy. Although the nurses had no problem transporting Elizabeth, sometimes accessing diagnostic areas may require special equipment for transportation. As with Elizabeth, the means to transfer heavier patients onto equipment or the equipment itself may not accommodate the patients' weight or girth. Diagnostic/procedural areas, such as radiology, physical therapy, and laboratory, should be notified as soon as the patient's physician orders are written. A minimum of at least one hour must be anticipated for scheduled procedures so they are able to assign an appropriate room for the bariatric patient. Ensure that the patient's weight and girth are measured and recorded prior to the scheduled test.

based on specific criteria. In managing the complex needs of the bariatric patient, preplanning for equipment has been thought to be the first step for intervention; however, it simply is not enough. Rather, a comprehensive interdisciplinary patient care approach may be necessary, and should include 1) a bariatric task force, 2) a criteria-based protocol, which includes preplanning for size-appropriate equipment, 3) a

competencies/skill set, and 4) outcome measurement efforts.

The value of an interdisciplinary bariatric task force as the initial phase of planning cannot be overlooked. The bariatric task force is an interdisciplinary quality improvement effort comprises interested and diverse parties from a variety of disciplines. The task force is designed to address ongoing issues and ideas and can

## PSYCHOSOCIAL ISSUES OF THE BARIATRIC PATIENT

**W**illiam and Timothy both have BMIs close to 60, which is where their similarities end. William is a minister of a popular Baptist Church, coaches high school basketball, and works at the local food bank. He loves himself as does his community; William has never given much thought to his body weight. Timothy, on the other hand, feels very conspicuous about his very heavy body. He reports he can't attend church, movies, or concerts because he simply doesn't fit properly in standard-sized chairs. He works full-time and otherwise spends most of his time at home. He openly states he despises his body, himself, and his life. William and Timothy are likely to respond differently emotionally when hospitalized. Typically, hospitalized patients report a lack of privacy and a loss of control. Unfamiliar surroundings can further lead to injuries and other problems. The obese patient, especially patients like Timothy, may be reluctant to accept physical care, can be difficult to assess, or may even refuse physical assessment because of embarrassment. The patient may have many issues related to a past experience in healthcare or a prolonged hospitalization. From an emotional perspective, each patient should be addressed individually because, although a person may be described as obese, they may or may not be affected emotionally by their weight. Patients like Timothy who express negative feelings about obesity and their body weight should be offered support in the form of a social services consult or chaplain consult depending on needs. Families may also need to be offered support. Staff could support the patient and/or family in the form of listening, discussing concerns, and offering suggestions. And whether caring for patients like William or like Timothy, it is inappropriate to refer to anyone by his or her weight or size. It is a violation of privacy statement to speak about a patient's size or weight with other staff members not involved in care.  Staff must be aware of their own feelings and opinions about obesity and its effect on patient care. Preplanning for care must include provision for emotional support based on the patient's actual needs.

include pharmacists, physical/occupational and respiratory therapists, physicians, clinical nurse specialists, ET/WOC nurses, and others. The inclusion of a patient representative is essential in that he or she understands the lived experience of being a larger, heavier patient. Each member of the team brings a unique and important perspective.[10]

Hospitals and other healthcare facilities should have a plan in place for the special needs of the morbidly obese patient. This can include equipment or clinical expert resources. A criteria-based protocol is simply preplanning based on specifically designated criteria.[11] The patient's weight, BMI, body width, and clinical condition serve as such criteria.

Actual weight is an important consideration in the weight limit of equipment, because if exceeded, then breakage, failure to function properly, or patient/caregiver injury can occur. Body width is described as the patient's body at his or her widest point, which could be at the patient's hips, shoulders, or across the belly when sidelying. Any clinical condition that interferes with mobility, such as pain, sedation, fear, or resistance to participate in care, places the patient at risk. Criteria-based protocols should be designed to meet the needs of the patient by ensuring access to specialty equipment and clinical experts in a timely, cost-effective manner.

Part of the preplanning effort must include provision for communication. Although sometimes difficult to arrange, a face to face interdisciplinary conference, which is planned within 24 hours of admission, may prevent costly intervention later.[12] Consider including the patient and his or her significant other, as this offers

## ROLE OF THE PT/OT IN COMATOSE, CRITICAL CARE PATIENTS

**K**aren is a 39-year-old, otherwise healthy woman with a body mass index (BMI )of 51. She fell while snowboarding and broke her ankle. Her treatment was provided by a hospital that cared for very few obese patients because of its proximity to the ski slopes. Most would agree that this hospital primarily dealt with orthopedic patients, 15 to 50 years old, with a mean BMI of 32. The hospital was ill prepared to manage Karen, and one issue led to another. On Day 3 in critical care, Karen was still medicated heavily and unable to walk or even reposition herself. The facility had no preplanning strategy for heavier patients, but the clinical staff began to have concerns about Karen's length of stay. In this particular setting, the physical therapist/occupational therapist (PT/OT) generally works with young, strong, orthopedic patients in helping them learn mobility techniques with the intent of discharge. Karen posed numerous other issues. The critical care unit held a team conference and discovered that the nurses and others were very concerned with their own safety in caring for Karen, and also the threat of deconditioning was mounting. The physical therapist, however, was experienced and educated to evaluate patients like Karen for strength, functional mobility, and safety issues, with the focus to prevent deconditioning. In coordinating preplanning efforts, it is imperative to include the PT/OT as the resource to manage these specific needs and others.

## PHARMACY

**S**everal factors alter pharmacokinetics among obese individuals. This can be due to fat distribution, protein binding, metabolism, and elimination of pharmaceutical agents. Resources and experts in this area are limited, and comprehensive drug dosage guides are not available to address this issue. Preplanning for care ought to include a clinical pharmacist to review the medication profiles on admission and throughout the hospital experience.

insight into the patient's special needs. Documentation of meetings, individual patient care goals, and corresponding intervention improves consistency and accountability. This level of accountability more fully defines each clinician's responsibilities.

Education provided to ensure basic skills or competencies is imperative and has become a critical part of any care plan. Consider conducting a survey to determine the actual learning needs of clinicians. The value of a diverse, interdisciplinary

bariatric task force is that it serves to provide a pool of experts to develop lesson plans that education clinicians. For example, assuming clinicians are seeking information pertaining to sensitivity, a social worker, chaplain, nurse expert, and patient member of the task force could develop a one-hour module to teach these skills.

In order to ensure long-term success of a comprehensive bariatric program, it is essential to understand and participate in outcome studies. Cost, clinical, and satisfaction research can be conducted to measure the value of an organizational improvement effort. Studies that examine time from admission to discharge, equipment availability, expert consultant, and incidence of skin injury document, from a quality perspective, the value of a comprehensive bariatric care plan.

## PREPARING FOR THE FUTURE

Although attempts to reduce body weight are common among Americans, the prevalence of obesity has continued to increase since the 1980s. Considering that more than two-thirds of US adults are overweight, it is likely that issues of caring for the overweight patient will continue. In fact, what is even more concerning is that not only has the percentage of overweight adult Americans increased, but the number of overweight children has doubled. And even though some overweight people are able to lose some of their body weight, a majority regain that weight within five years.[13]

Such increases will adversely affect healthcare delivery systems since obesity is strongly associated with several chronic diseases. This may lead to costly hospitalization, especially in the absence of preplanning. Recent estimates suggest that obesity-related morbidity currently accounts for 6.8 percent of US healthcare costs.[14] This increasing prevalence will likely impact acute care and may not only influence the frequency of admission, but will influence the severity of care that the patients of the future will require when hospitalized. Clinicians best serve the needs of the patient and their organizations when policies and protocols are in place to guide preplanning for the care. Continued use of interdisciplinary teams is essential to more fully understand the interdepartmental impact of caring for overweight patients in the

## IMPLICATIONS FOR DISCHARGE

The bariatric patient needs to be referred to a case manager or social worker for continuity of care and discharge planning. The designated case manager/social worker will interview the patient for needs. The case manager/social worker will determine the payer source and inform the appropriate physicians and team members which financial resources are available as it relates to continued stay and discharge. The case manager/social worker will consult with nursing, PT/OT, and others to determine the patient's needs and to acquire equipment. If the patient is a candidate for rehabilitation, a referral may be made to an appropriate facility. If a referral is made to a facility that does not have bariatric equipment, the accepting facility needs enough time to order the needed equipment. All referrals are made according to payer source. Nursing is responsible for providing patient/family teaching regarding skin care. The patient or their caregiver must be assessed for their ability to apply topical creams, medications, and dressings. If the patient is to be transferred to rehab, the weight of the patient must be communicated to the transporter. If the patient is going home and needs special equipment at home, the case manager/social worker can serve as a resource. The wound care specialist may also be able to assist in locating equipment. When home health is involved, be sure home health knows this is a bariatric patient.

## IDEAS FOR BARIATRIC EQUIPMENT

- Ambulatory/mobility aids: Transfer bench, trapeze, hover-type lateral transfer, slide sheet, lift and transfer product, walker, wheelchair, stretcher, reclining wheelchair
- Bathing/bathroom: Commode, bedpan, shower chair, handheld shower
- Beds: Frame, support surface
- Others: Blood pressure cuff, diapers, drape/gowns, diagnostic equipment, scales, tables, binders, surgical instruments, tracheostomy tubes, tube holders

acute care setting. Furthermore, manufacturers and vendors need clinical input in order to more fully understand the unique equipment needs of the larger patient.

Solutions to this industry-wide problem are not simple. The challenge to hospitals and caregivers is that all these changes must be done in a growing climate where profit and reductions outweigh caregiver safety and patient care.[15]

## CONCLUSION

With obesity on the rise, wound care clinicians are increasingly responsible for managing the needs of this complex patient population. Although preplanning for equipment is a helpful adjunct to care, it is never a substitute for care. Numerous resources are available to clinicians across practice settings, and use of resources in a timely and appropriate manner are thought to improve measurable therapeutic, satisfaction, and cost outcomes. Coordinating these resources in the form of a comprehensive bariatric care plan may ensure the most favorable outcome. The obese patient holds numerous care challenges, and it is in the interest of healthcare organizations to meet these skin and wound care challenges in a clinically, ethically, and legally sound manner.[16]

## REFERENCES

1.  Medical care for obese patients: Advise for health care professional. National Task Force on the Prevention and Treatment of Obesity. *Am Fam Physician* 2002;65:81–8.
2.  Kral J. Morbid obesity and related health risks. *Ann Int Med* 1985;103(6 part 2): 1043–7.
3.  Gallagher SM. Meeting the needs of the obese patient. *AJN* 1996;96(8)supp:1s–12s.
4.  Charney W. An epidemic of health care worker injury. In: William Charney, Guy Fragala (eds). *An Epidemic of Health Care Worker Injury: An Epidemiology.* New York: CRC Press, 1998.
5.  Gallagher S. Caring for the overweight patient in the acute care setting: addressing caregiver injury. *J Healthcare, Safety, Compliance, and Infection Control* 200:4(8):379–82.
6.  Gallagher S. Understanding barriers to protocol development. National WOCN conference: Las Vegas NV, 2002.
7.  Gallagher SM. Outcomes in clinical practice: Pressure ulcers prevalence and incidence studies. *Ost Wound Manage* 1997;43(1):28–40.
8.  Gallagher SM. Morbid obesity: A chronic disease with an impact on wounds and related problems. *Ost Wound Manage* 1997;45(5):18–27.
9.  Gallagher SM. Restructuring the therapeutic environment to promote care and safety for the obese patient. JWOCN 1999;26:292–7.
10.  Gallagher S. Bariatrics: Considering mobility, patient safety, and caregiver injury. In: Charney W, Hudson A. *Back Injury Among Healthcare Workers.* Baton Rouge, LA: Lewis Publishers, 2004.
11.  Gallagher S. Restructuring the therapeutic environment to promote care and safety for the obese patient. *JWOCN* 1999;26:292–7.
12.  DeRuiter HP, Meitteunen E, Sauder K. Improving safety for caregivers through collaborative practice. *J Heathcare Safety, Compliance, and Infection Control* 2001;5(2):61–64.
13.  Yanovski JA, Yanovski SZ. Recent advances in basic obesity research. *J Am Med Assoc* 1999;282(16):1504–6.
14.  Wolf AM, Coditz GA. Social and economic effects of body weight in the United States. *Am J Clin Nutr* 1996;53:1595s–603s.
15.  Charney W. An epidemic of health care worker injury. In: William Charney, Guy Fragala. An epidemic of health care worker injury: An epidemiology. New York, NY: CRC Press, 1998.
16.  Gallagher SM. Morbid obesity: A chronic disease with an impact on wounds and related problems. *Ost Wound Manage* 1997;45(5):18–27.

# 18

# Writing for Publication

**C**ommunicating to colleagues is an important professional practice responsibility. Poster presentations, oral presentations, and published articles all serve to share information. Selecting a topic, researching it, and organizing it into a suitable method for communicating are discussed, whether the work is prepared for a unit-based oral presentation, a professional journal article, or a national poster presentation. A detailed description to getting started is discussed, with timelines, key words for the literature search, key journals and groups soliciting information, writing the query letter, grammar and style, rejection and revisions, and strategies for staying enthused.

Most writers have some idea of what interests them, and therefore selecting a topic is usually easy. Successful writers write about subjects they feel passionate about, have an interest in, or a commitment to. Ask yourself, "What do I enjoy reading about and talking about? What patients do I find most interesting?"

**FOR MORE INFORMATION**

**Interested in more information on finding an appropriate journal, submission guidelines, referencing guides, and more, please see:**

**http://www.library.jhu.edu/researchhelp/general/publishing.html**
**http://members.aol.com/suzannehj/naed.htm**

The next step to identifying a topic is to select a topic specific enough to ensure the content can be covered well. Successful authors work from general to specific or specific to general. For example, consider the problem of unsuspected anastomic leak post-BWLS. In moving from general to specific, consider the following thought progression. Although it is a very important topic, is it too broad? What could be covered? Who is at risk? What are the cardinal signs? How does one communicate findings with the surgeon? Does it matter if the leak is early or late postoperatively? Or maybe the writer wants to focus on what might be called information gaps. Most clinicians understand sepsis, and widespread infection, so why is anastomotic leak frequently missed when it comes to the obese patient? Is there an information gap? What about an article that addresses the specific challenges to assessment?

Once a topic has been selected, begin talking to clinical experts and members of the target audience. Who will read your article? Who will listen to your lecture? Who is interested in your poster? If the target journal is *Critical Care Nurse*, interview nurses who read that particular journal. In writing about obstructive sleep apnea in the intensive care unit, consider talking with critical care nurses. Who are the patients? What are their families like? How do nurses feel about taking care of the obese patient with respiratory compromise? What are the real world challenges inherent in caring for this parent population? Are the issues intubation, extubation, skin care, tracheostomy care, secretion control, family issues, or something else? Once the writer has determined the real-world issues, he or she should interview clinical experts. Find out if the clinical experts find the topic interesting enough to attend a lecture on it or to read about it in a journal. Talk with experts across disciplines, settings, and institutions. Using the above example, consider a pulmonologist, sleep center clinician, respiratory therapist, nurse expert, or equipment vendor at a number of different institutions. Most clinicians are willing to share, especially if the author designates a time to talk and gives a limit on the amount of time needed. For example, the writer can ask, "Can we talk for 20 minutes Thursday at 10:00am to discuss obstructive sleep apnea in the critical care unit from a pulmonologist's perspective?"

Once the writer has selected a topic and interviewed members of the target audience and clinical experts, a literature review can be done. Use words, phrases, and associated conditions that were discussed with those interviewed. Perhaps CPAP, BiPAP, trach tube holder, rotation therapy, Portex trach tube, and elevated intra-abdominal pressure need to be investigated further. A medical librarian is especially helpful. Understand what the term *key words* means in a literature search. Consider a Boolean search in grouping words together to find meaningful literature. Seek current literature, historic literature, and information published in the popular magazines and newspapers. Keep in mind, however, that the more stringent the source's review process, the more meaningful the literature. Therefore, many interesting, popular magazine, newspapers, and tabloids are considered the least reliable sources.

Once the literature has been collected, reviewed, and categorized, the outline can be developed. There are at least two ways to prepare an outline. These two popular styles are sometimes referred to as *left brain outline* and *right brain outline*. The left brain outline is a more traditional, orderly style of outline using the following:
1. Title
2. Problem/Purpose/Goal
3. Hypothesis
4. References
5. Opportunities.

The right brain outline has been helpful for anyone with writer's block. Some writers plot out both styles and then prepare the manuscript or lecture from there. A right brain outline is truly brainstorming. The very first step in this type of outline is to close out the left brain, put those organized thoughts away, and allow the right brain to do what it does best, which is to be creative. Authors report that this process can be a lot of fun if done right. Relax, get out colored paper and pens, and begin to write down thoughts quickly, paying no attention to grammar or spelling. Similar thoughts should be

placed on the paper close to one another, but not linearly like a left brain outline.

In finalizing a topic, target audience, and method of delivery, take a few minutes and review all of the research thus far. Ask the questions posed earlier. Barriers in this final process of planning are a topic that is too broad or a target audience that has just published/heard a similar topic. A query letter will resolve these issues whether you are writing to a coordinator of a conference interested in the lecture/poster or an editor interested in the article. Interest in the topic does not guarantee acceptance, but most editors/coordinators will share if the topic is not appropriate, suitable, or timely.

## PUNCTUATION

Punctuation is the road map to written clarity. Different styles of punctuation are based on different situations. Readers should never have to reread for

understanding. The period, exclamation point, dash, semicolon, colon, contraction, and paragraph are all important in guiding the reader to understand the meaning of the written words. The period signals the end of a sentence, and is the most common way to end a sentence in academic work. The exclamation point signals excitement, which is not necessarily appropriate for an academic presentation. The reader should feel enthusiasm by reading interpretation or explanation of the research/work. For example, "The results of this study are staggering," is not necessary if the writing instead states, "The team saw a 100-percent decrease in infection rate over the six-month period of time." No exclamation point is necessary in that statement; any clinician feels the excitement and wants more information. Also, readers will understand that the results are staggering.

The dash can be used as a

**ADDITIONAL READING**

Mee C. *10 Lessons on Writing for Publication.* Author guidelines and writing tips. Available at:www.nursing2004.com

Lukeman N. *The First Five Pages: A Writers' Guide to Staying Out of the Rejection Pile.* New York, NY: Simon Schuster, 2000.

Zinsser W. *On Writing Well: the Classic Guide to Writing Nonfiction.* New York, NY: Harper Collins, 2001.

substitute for a comma, especially when the writer wants to add intrigue or variety to a paper where appropriate. The semicolon is used to signal the reader to read on for more related information when either *for, and, nor, but, yet,* or *so* (FANBOYS) are not used to link two otherwise complete thoughts. For example: "The application deadline for magnet status was September 3; we will apply for an extension." The colon can be used two ways. The first is a command to read on for further explanation of a primary thought. For example: "We can trace the pressure ulcer to one cause: failure to turn the patient." The second use of the colon is to list examples: "We can more accurately trace the pressure ulcer to several factors: failure to turn the patient, unrelieved pressure on the OR table, and poor hydration." Contractions such as *can't, don't,* or *couldn't* are used in informal writing and speaking; they are seldom used in academic or professional presentations.

A paragraph is a structure in writing that follows one complete thought. The distinction of a bridging paragraph is that it has an opening and closing sentence, with two to three sentences in between. A power paragraph has a key sentence and

## REJECTION/REVISION

Eighty percent of manuscripts are rejected. Keep that in mind when submitting. As soon as the manuscript is submitted to the journal of choice, begin looking for an alternative. The manuscript can only be submitted to one journal at a time, and the time period for review may be six months, but in that time, think about other options. Review the alternative's submission guidelines for referencing and any other changes that might have to be made before submitting to the second choice, but be prepared. Many great articles sit in the body of the computer because the first choice journal had just accepted a manuscript of a similar topic, and there wasn't room for both. The same holds for revisions, except that nearly 100 percent of manuscripts will require revision. Rather than seeing this as a deficiency, recognize that the revision process is the "home stretch" to publication. A hint that makes revisions more tolerable is to have all of the interviews, outlines, documentation, files, and references in one place. No one wants to do the research twice, and most authors agree that by revision time the author may be weary of what was once a very exciting topic. Do not delay on revisions, because an equally great manuscript of a similar topic may be waiting on the editor's desk. If there is a delay, call the editor and discuss the status. Communication is critical at this point in the process.

## POSTER PRESENTATION

Poster presentations are exciting methods of communicating information. Many journal editors attend poster sessions looking for potential manuscript authors. Every conference seems to have different guidelines for poster presentations, and within the guidelines there can be different categories for submission. For example, there might be categories such as *professional practice, case study,* or *original research* all within the same set of submission guidelines. Poster presentations generally feature *recently completed, not yet published in a journal, types of research, case study(ies)* or *projects.* These presentations are usually very timely. Look to the conference information website for detailed submission guidelines and deadlines, and call the coordinator for specific questions. Take care to read the guidelines carefully and follow them exactly. Don't allow complex guidelines be discouraging, as poster presentations can lead to a journal article or other opportunity to share important information.

a thesis statement. Paragraphs are usually four typewritten lines, but there is flexibility in this. Be aware that readers may get lost in an especially long paragraph unless it is very well written.

Once the manuscript is

## GETTING STARTED

**Find an honest, encouraging colleague or friend.**
**Select an exciting topic.**
**Make the commitment.**
**Sustain momentum.**

## WRITING IS NOT AN ART

**Writing is not an art; it is practice, failure, practice, less failure, practice, etc. Use a written style that conveys your personality. Use your written voice. Convey personal warmth and spirit. Let your written voice assert confidence in yourself, your knowledge, and your expert skill. Avoid verbal clutter; be aware of long, unnecessarily complicated words. Avoid prepositions, and be prepared to prune, prune, prune. Be aware of the trend to use nouns as adjectives, adjectives as nouns, and nouns as verbs. Consider the evolution of words, and to create a classic, timeless work, avoid verbal fads and trends. For example, use of *bad, hot, cool, chill, awesome*, and other expressions will date your work and confuse your reader.**

written, expect to take an equal amount of time with the proofing and editing. With that being said, remember that the manuscript does not have to be perfect, as perfection is a relative term, but it needs to be clear enough that the editor can follow the meaning of the paper without a reread. Spell and grammar checks are useful tools, but only tools. For example, this statement was discovered in a college paper addressing courtesy in the clinical setting, "The physician showed curtsies to his patients." Spellchecking is never a substitute for good proofreading.

Proofreading is an important skill. When doing final proofing, read the entire manuscript out loud, ask a friend who is outside of your professional area to read the manuscript, and focus on one line at a time. When statements are made, constantly remind yourself to ask why. For example, suppose the statement reads, "Pressure-related skin injury can occur between skin folds in the intertriginous regions among hospitalized patients." The editor will want an explanation to why. The statement more accurately reads, "Pressure-related skin injury can occur between skin folds in the intertriginous regions among hospitalized patients because interface pressures can exceed 32mm pressure within the folds." For each statement made, consider completing it by answering the *why* question.

Control for errors by keeping references together and readily available. Know the content in the references, and if there is a question as to what an author intended to say in a published article that is being referenced, call the author to clarify. Keep a reference guide, style guide, and thesaurus close by.

## FINDING SUCCESS

Control the fear of rejection; keep in mind that manuscripts are rejected for many reasons, not necessarily because of content or writing style. If it is unclear why the manuscript is rejected, call the editor and prepare to listen and ask questions. Consider the question, "What journal might be interested in this manuscript?" Remember only 20 percent of manuscripts are accepted at first submission, and revisions are not rejections. The greatest threat to publication is procrastination. Before thinking about publication, decide whether the time is right for you. Some authors find that sharing the responsibility with a coauthor is motivating and keeps them on track, and others feel it interferes. Each author must determine his or her unique style and when the time is right, and pursue this opportunity to that extent.

## BLOCKING WRITERS' BLOCK

Everyone suffers from writers' block at one time or another. Good writers realize that writing is a job, and those who wait to be inspired will probably never complete the project. Some writers will write for an allocated period of time every day regardless of the way they feel that day. Yet, what can be done when the block sets in? Some suggest that a manuscript can be written from the "inside out." Who says writing needs to begin with an introduction? Once the goal and objections of the manuscript have been established, there are no rules regarding order in which the paper should be written. Think about the right brain outline, locate the categories of thought, and work from there. Any time the writer finds that three minutes have passed without a word on the page, it might be time to find a new page.

## SAMPLE QUERY LETTER

Your Name and Credentials
Mailing Address
City, State Zip
Phone Number
E-mail Address

Editor's Name and Title/Credentials
Journal Name
Address
City State Zip

August 28, 2006

Dear Ms Smith:

Little has been published regarding the complexities of wound care, pulmonary issues, and obesity. As a critical care nurse and member of the Bariatric Task Force here at St John's Medical Center, I am aware of the complex nursing needs of this particular patient population.

I believe readers of Journal Name would find the article I am planning of interest in their everyday care of critically ill patients in that the number of obese patients with obstructive sleep apnea and chronic/acute wounds has increased over 75% in the unit where I work. I believe this is probably the case nationwide.

The manuscript can be available December 1, 2006. Please let me know if Journal Name is interested.

Sincerely,

Your Signature

Your Name and Credentials
Phone Number
E-mail Address
Title
Employer
Employer Address

## SUMMARY

Writing for publication is simply a sharing process, a very important process in that information becomes available to hundreds and sometimes thousands of interested clinicians. Writing and sharing is valuable in many ways. The impact that one single clinician can make on the community of clinicians caring for obese patients is phenomenal. Patient care evolves and develops because of publication of pertinent research and information. Finally, the excitement of seeing one's name in print is staggering!

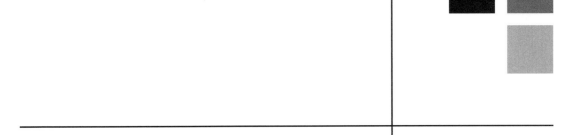

# Glossary of Terms

**ABG:** Arterial blood gas analysis.
**acrp30:** adipocyte complement-related protein of 30 kDa.
**Activities of daily living (ADLs):** Activities routinely performed daily by the average person in a given society.
**Adipocyte:** Fat cell.
**Adipose:** The fat present in the cells of adipose tissue.
**Adiposity:** Obesity.
**ADLs:** Activities of daily living.
**Agency for Health Care Policy and Research (AHCPR):** This agency has been renamed Agency for Healthcare Research and Quality.
**Agency for Health Care Research and Quality (AHRQ):** An agency that is part of the United States Department of Health and Human Services with the mission of improving the quality, safety, efficiency, and effectiveness of healthcare for all Americans.
**AHCPR:** Agency for Health Care Policy and Research, this agency has been renamed Agency for Healthcare Research and Quality.
**AHRQ:** Agency for Healthcare Research and Quality.
**Albumin:** A protein made in the liver that assists in maintaining blood volume in the arteries and veins.
**Aldosterone:** The major miner-alocorticoid secreted by the adrenal cortex; it promotes retention of sodium and bicar-

bonate, excretion of potassium and hydrogen ions, and secondary retention of water.

**Alveolus:** Anatomic nomenclature for a small saclike structure, especially in the jaws or lungs.

**American Society for Bariatric Surgery (ASBS):** Founded in 1983, this organization seeks to provide educational and support programs and advance the art and science of bariatric surgery for surgeons and allied health professionals in the field of bariatrics.

**Amphetamine:** Racemic amphetamine, (±)-_ methylphenethylamine, a sympathomimetic amine that has a stimulating effect on both the central and peripheral nervous systems. It relaxes both systolic and diastolic blood pressure and bronchial muscle, contracts the sphincter of the urinary bladder, and depresses the appetite.

**Anorexia nervosa:** An eating disorder characterized by refusal to maintain a normal minimal body weight, intense fear of gaining weight or becoming obese, a disturbance of body image resulting in a feeling of being fat or having fat in certain areas even when extremely emaciated, undue reliance on body weight or shape for self-evaluation, and amenorrhea.

**Antimicrobial:** An agent that kills microorganisms or suppresses their multiplication or growth.

**Appetite:** Natural longing or desire, especially the natural and recurring desire for food.

**Arterial blood gas analysis (ABG):** The analysis of the partial pressures of oxygen and carbon dioxide in blood.

**ASBS:** American Society for Bariatric Surgery.

**Atelectasis:** Incomplete expansion of a lung or a portion of a lung; it may be a primary (congenital), secondary, or otherwise acquired condition.

**Bardet-Biedl syndrome:** An autosomal recessive disorder characterized by mental retardation, pigmentary retinopathy, obesity, polydactyly, and hypogonadism.

**Bariatric weight loss surgery (BWLS):** Surgical management of obesity, including laparoscopic Roux-en-Y gastric bypass [RNYGB], open RNYGB, laparoscopic banding, balloon, etc.

**Bariatrics:** The study of overweight, its causes, prevention, and treatment.

**Biliopancreatic diversion (BPD):** A portion of the stomach is removed and the remaining portion of the stomach is connected to the lower portion of small intestine.

**Esophagitis:** Inflammation of the esophagus.

**BATOS:** Bray Attitude Toward Obesity Survey.

**Beneficence:** The act of doing good.

**Biguanides:** Any of a group of substituted deriatives of biguanide, which are used as oral antihyperglycemic agents; they increase insulin action in peripheral tissues and by inhibiting gluconeogenesis decrease hepatic glucose production.

**BMI:** Body mass index.

**Body mass index (BMI):** The weight in kilograms divided by the square of the height in meters, a measure of body fat that gives an indication of nutritional status.

**BPD:** Biliopancreatic diversion.

**Bray Attitude Toward Obesity Survey (BATOS):** A 40-item, Likert, easily scored, self-assessment tool designed to measure attitudes toward obesity among all areas of specialty or discipline.

**Bulimia:** Episodic binge eating usually followed by behavior designed to negate the excessive caloric intake, most commonly purging behaviors such as self-induced vomiting or laxative abuse but sometimes other methods, such as excessive exercise or fasting. While it is usually associated with bulimia nervosa, it may also occur in other disorders, such as anorexia nervosa.

**BWLS:** Bariatric weight loss surgery.

**Calorie:** A unit of measurement that specifies the energy content of foods.

***Candida albicans:*** A species that is part of the normal flora of human skin and mucous membranes and is the most frequent cause of candidiasis.

**Candidiasis:** Infection with a fungus of the genus Candida, especially *C. albicans*. It is usually a superficial infection of the skin or mucous membranes, although sometimes it manifests as a systemic infection or endocarditis; any form can become more severe in immunocompromised patients.

**Catecholamine:** One of a group

of biogenic amines having a sympathomimetic action, the aromatic portion of whose molecule is catechol, and the aliphatic portion an amine; examples are dopamine, norepinephrine, and epinephrine.

**CDT:** Complete decongestive therapy.

**Cellulitis:** An acute, diffuse, spreading, edematous, suppurative inflammation of the deep subcutaneous tissues and sometimes muscle, sometimes with abscess formation. It is usually caused by infection of a wound, burn, or other cutaneous lesion by bacteria, especially group A streptococci and *Staphylococcus aureus*, but it may also occur in immunocompromised hosts or following erysipelas.

**Chronic respiratory acidosis:** Respiratory acidosis occurs when the lungs cannot remove all of the carbon dioxide (a normal by-product of metabolism) produced by the body. This causes a disturbance of the acid-base balance in which body fluids become excessively acidic.

**Circumgastric banding:** Stomach size is limited by an inflatable band placed around the fundus of the stomach. The band is connected to a subcutaneous port and can be inflated or deflated (by fluid injection in the healthcare provider's office) to change the stoma size to meet the patient's needs as she loses weight. Banding can be done laparoscopically.

**CLRT:** Continuous lateral rotation therapy.

**Colostomy:** The surgical creation of an opening between the colon and the surface of the body; also used to refer to the opening, or stoma, so created.

**Complete decongestive therapy (CDT):** A noninvasive treatment used as a rehabilitative intervention for chronic intractable lymphedema. The objective of the technique is to redirect and enhance the flow of lymph through intact cutaneous lymphatics.

**Congestive heart failure (CHF):** A clinical syndrome due to heart disease, characterized by breathlessness and abnormal sodium and water retention, often resulting in edema.

**Continuous lateral rotation therapy (CLRT):** Turning the patient less than 40 degrees along a longitudinal axis.

**Continuous positive airway pressure (CPAP):** A method of positive pressure ventilation used with patients who are breathing spontaneously, in which pressure in the airway is maintained above the level of atmospheric pressure throughout the respiratory cycle. The purpose is to keep the alveoli open at the end of exhalation and thus increase oxygenation and reduce the work of breathing.

**CPAP:** Continuous positive airway pressure.

**Criteria-based protocol:** Preplanning based on specifically designated criteria.

**Curves for Women:** National fitness franchise for women that consists of a 30-minute exercise program along with weightloss guidance.

**Debridement:** The removal of foreign material and dead or damaged tissue from the wound bed.

**Deep vein thrombosis (DVT):** Formation of blood clots in the deep veins of the legs and pelvis. People recovering from abdominal surgery are at increased risk for these clots, as are overweight individuals.

**Dermis:** The layer of the skin deep to the epidermis, consisting of a dense bed of vascular connective tissue.

**Duodenal switch:** This is a variation of BPD that leaves a larger portion of the stomach intact, including the pyloric valve that regulates the release of stomach contents into the small intestine. It also keeps a small part of the duodenum in the digestive pathway.

**Dumping syndrome:** A group of symptoms that occur when food or liquid enters the small intestine too rapidly. These symptoms include cramps, nausea, diarrhea, and dizziness. Dumping syndrome sometimes occurs in people who have had a portion of their stomach removed.

**Duodenum:** The first or proximal portion of the small intestine, extending from the pylorus to the jejunum; so called because it is about 12 fingerbreadths in length.

**DVT:** Deep vein thrombosis.

**Dyslipoproteinemia:** The presence of abnormal concentrations of lipoproteins, or of abnormal lipoproteins, in the blood.

**Enteric:** Of intestinal origin, especially applied to wastes or bacteria.

**Epidermis:** The outermost and nonvascular layer of the skin, derived from the embryonic ectoderm, varying in thickness from 0.07 to 0.12 mm, except on the palms and soles where it may be 0.8 and 1.4 mm, respectively.

**Epithelization (epithelialization):** Healing by the growth of epithelium over a denuded surface.

**Ergonomics:** The science relating to humans and their work, embodying the anatomic, physiologic, psychologic, and mechanical principles affecting the efficient use of human energy.

**Ethics (medical):** The values and guidelines that should govern decisions in medicine.

**Evidence-based practice:** Clinical decision-making based on a systematic review of the scientific evidence of the risks, benefits, and costs of alternative forms of diagnosis or treatment

**Expiratory reserve volume:** The largest amount of air that can be forced out of the lungs after a normal breath has already been breathed out.

**FBLRT:** Full-body lateral rotation.

**Fen-phen:** An anti-obesity medication (an anorectic) that consisted of fenfluramine and phentermine.

**FRC:** Functional residual capacity.

**Functional residual capacity (FRC):** This is the lung volume at the end of a normal expiration, when the muscles of respiration are completely relaxed; at FRC and at FRC only, the tendency of the lungs to collapse is exactly balanced by the tendency of the chest wall to expand.

**Gastric restriction and malabsorption surgery:** Also known as gastric bypass or Roux-en-Y gastric bypass, the procedure creates a small stomach pouch with an anastomosis to the jejunum. Food the patient eats bypasses 90% of the stomach, the duodenum, and a limb of jejunum of varying length, so fewer calories are absorbed. This procedure also can be performed laparoscopically.

**Gastroesophageal reflux disease (GERD):** The movement of food, fluids, and digestive juices from the stomach back up into the esophagus; causes irritation of the esophagus with acid, resulting in discomfort. GERD occurs when the muscle between the stomach and the esophagus, known as the lower esophageal sphincter, opens when it should stay closed, or is weak.

**Gastrointestinal:** Pertaining to or communicating with the stomach and intestine. Called also enterogastric and gastroenteric.

**Gene polymorphism:** A trait of an organism that is found in more than one state in a population. Also used for the existence of different forms of a gene in a population. For example, one well known polymorphism of color vision is the existence of both red-green dichromats and normal trichromats in the human population.

**Georgetown Mantra:** Consists of four principles: autonomy,

beneficence, non-maleficence, and justice.

**GERD:** Gastroesophageal reflux disease.

**Growth factors:** Small proteins produced by the human body that enable cells to communicate and effectively coordinate activities between one another.

**Gynecoid obesity:** Fat distribution in a female fashion.

**Hydrocolloid:** A waterproof, occlusive dressing that consists of a mixture of pectins, gelatins, sodium carboxymethylcellulose, and elastomers.

**Hydrogel:** A dressing that comes as a sheet or gel with a high water content, which aids the rehydration of hard eschar and promotes autolysis in necrotic wounds.

**Hydrotherapy:** A daily bathing used to clean the wound and soften eschar in order to aid in the healing process.

**Hyperinsulinemia:** Refers to high levels of insulin in the blood, frequently resulting from insulin resistance.

**Hyperlipidemia:** A general term for elevated concentrations of any or all of the lipids in the plasma, such as hypertriglyceridemia and hypercholesterolemia.

**Hypersomnolence (hypersomnia):** Excessive sleeping or sleepiness, as in any of a group of sleep disorders with a variety of physical and psychogenic causes.

**Hypopnea:** Episode of decreased rate and depth of breathing.

**Hypoventilation syndrome (Pickwickian syndrome):** A condition related to (but can occur separately from) obstructive sleep apnea. In OHS, a very obese person does not breathe a sufficient amount of oxygen during sleep or while awake.

**IAT:** Implicit Association Test.

**Ileus:** Obstruction of the bowel; specifically a condition that is commonly marked by a painful distended abdomen, vomiting of dark or fecal matter, toxemia, and dehydration.

**IM:** Intramuscular.

**Implicit Association Test (IAT):** A method that demonstrates the conscious-unconscious divergences.

**Incontinence:** Loss of bladder and/or bowel control.

**Informed consent/refusal:** A person's voluntary agreement or refusal, based upon adequate knowledge and understanding of relevant information, to participate in research or to undergo a diagnostic, therapeutic, or preventive procedure. In giving informed consent, subjects may not waive or appear to waive any of their legal rights, or release or appear to release the investigator, the sponsor, the institution or agents thereof from liability for negligence.

**Intertrigo:** Inflammatory dermatosis caused by skin rubbing against skin coupled with heat and moisture.

**Intramuscular (IM):** To give a substance through an injection into muscle tissue.

**Intrathecal:** Injection into the innermost membrane surrounding the central nervous system. Usually done by lumbar puncture.

**Intravenous (IV):** Of or pertaining to the inside of a vein, as of a thrombus. An injection made directly into a vein.

**IV:** Intravenous.

**JCAHCO:** Joint Commission on Accreditation of Healthcare Organizations.

**Jejunum:** The second portion of the small intestine extending from the duodenum to the ileum.

**Joint Commission on Accreditation of Healthcare Organizations (JCAHCO):** The Joint Commission is an independent, not-for-profit organization, established more than 50 years ago. Joint Commission is governed by a board that includes physicians, nurses, and consumers. Joint Commission sets the standards by which health care quality is measured in America and around the world.

**Laparoscopic gastric banding:** A minimally invasive procedure in which a band is placed around the stomach, which restricts the stomach size and allows the patient to lose weight by creating a sense of fullness and preventing the patient from consuming large amounts of food.

**LAP-BAND®:** Trade name for laparoscopic gastric banding procedure.

**Laurence-Moon-Biedl syndrome:** An autosomal recessive condition characterized by mental retardation, retinitis pigmentosa, hypogonadism, spastic paraplegia, obesity, polydactyly, cataract, squint, and renal anomalies (calyceal cysts, clubbing or diverticula; fetal lobulation)

**Leptin:** A protein hormone that helps regulate body weight, metabolism, and reproductive function.

**Lipedema:** Chronic swelling, usually of the lower extremities, caused by widespread, even distribution of subcutaneous fat and fluid.

**Lipolysis:** The increased fat breakdown in the body tissues that occurs in ketosis (lysis of fat).

**Lymphedema:** A condition in which excess fluid collects in tissue and causes swelling. It may occur in the arm or leg after lymph vessels or lymph nodes in the underarm or groin are blocked or removed.

**Lymphocyte:** A type of white blood cell that plays a number of roles in the immune system, including the production of antibodies and other substances that fight infection and diseases.

**Lipolysis:** The decomposition or splitting up of fat.

**Malabsorption:** The inability to adequately or efficiently absorb nutrients from the intestinal tract.

**Malnutrition:** Any disorder of nutrition causing a lack of necessary or proper food substances in the body or improper absorption and distribution of them.

**Metabolic syndrome:** A collection of metabolic risk factors in one individual. The root causes of metabolic syndrome are overweight/obesity, physical activity, and genetic factors. Various risk factors have been included in metabolic syndrome. Factors generally accepted as being characteristic of this syndrome include

abdominal obesity, athero-
genic dyslipidemia, raised
blood pressure, insulin resistance with or without glucose
intolerance, prothrombotic
state, and proinflammatory
state.

**Mortality:** The death rate or
the ratio of the total number
of deaths to the total population.

**Morbid obesity:** A disease in
which excess weight begins
to interfere with basic physiological functions, such as
breathing and walking.
Generally, it can be defined as
weighing 100 pounds more
than the ideal weight. A more
precise indicator is a BMI of
40 or greater.

**Morbidity:** Any departure, subjective or objective, from a
state of physiological or psychological well being. In this
sense, sickness, illness, and a
morbid condition are synony-
mous.

**NAAFA:** National Association to
Advance Fat Acceptance.

**Naloxone:** A drug that blocks
the pain alleviation ascribed
to endorphins and inhibits the
effect of morphine and similar
opiates by binding to opiate
receptors in the brain.

**National Association to
Advance Fat Acceptance
(NAAFA):** Founded in 1969,
the National Association to
Advance Fat Acceptance is a
non-profit human rights
organization dedicated to
improving the quality of life
for fat people. NAAFA works
to eliminate discrimination
based on body size and provide fat people with the tools
for self-empowerment
through public education,
advocacy, and member sup-
port.

**Necrosis:** Localized tissue
death.

**Nephrosis:** A condition caused
by failure of the kidneys to
cleanse the blood. If the kidneys cannot remove waste
products from the blood, the
waste products accumulate in
the bloodstream.

**Nosocomial:** Denoting a new
disorder (not the patient's
original condition) associated
with being treated in a hospital, such as a hospital-
acquired infection.

**OA:** Overeaters Anonymous.

**Obesity:** The condition in which
excess fat has accumulated in
the body; usually considered
to be 20 percent above the
recommended weight for
height and age, and a BMI of
30 or higher.

**Obesity hypoventilation syn-
drome (OHS):** A group of
symptoms characterized by
massive obesity, flushed face,
frequent short episodes of
irresistible sleep throughout
the day, and disturbed sleep
at night.

**Obstructive sleep apnea
(OSA):** A condition that
occurs during sleep when a
person stops breathing for 10
seconds or longer as a result
of blockage in the airway that
prevents air from getting to
the lungs.

**Occupational Safety and
Health Administration
(OSHA):** A Federal agency
under the Department of
Labor that publishes and
enforces safety and health
regulations for most business-
es and industries in the
United States.

**OHS:** Obesity hypoventilation
syndrome.

**Orlistat:** A commonly pre-
scribed fat absorption medication, it is sold under the
brand name Xenical.

**OSA:** Obstructive sleep apnea.

**OSHA:** Occupational Safety and
Health Administration.

**Osteoarthritis:** Arthritis characterized by erosion of articu-
lar cartilage, either primary or
secondary to trauma or other
conditions, which becomes
soft, frayed, and thinned with
eburnation of subchondral
bone and outgrowths of mar-
ginal osteophytes.

**Overeaters Anonymous (OA):**
A group support program
offering recovery from compulsive overeating using the
12 steps and 12 traditions as
interpreted by OA. Like other
12-step groups, OA groups
typically meet weekly.

**Overweight:** Being too heavy
for one's height. It is defined
as a body mass index (BMI)
of 25 up to 30kg/m².

**Panniculectomy:** The surgical
removal of excess tissue and
skin from the abdomen.

**Parenteral:** Administered intravenously or by injection.

**Paternalism:** The attitude (of a
person or a government) that
subordinates should be controlled in a fatherly way for
their own good.

**Peer review:** The process by
which articles are chosen to
be included in a refereed
journal. An editorial board
consisting of experts in the
same field as the author
review the article and decide
if it is authoritative enough
for publication.

**Phentermine:** An appetite suppressant that disrupts the transmission of signals from the neurotransmitters and is used in the management of obesity.

**Plasma renin activity:** Also called plasma renin assay, may be used to screen for high blood pressure (hypertension) of kidney origin, and may help plan treatment of essential hypertension, a genetic disease often aggravated by excess sodium intake.

**Prader-Willi Syndrome:** A genetic disorder of chromosome 15 marked by hypotonia, short stature, hyperphagia, cognitive impairment, poor feeding and growth in infancy, and when not carefully managed, characterized by obesity.

**Pressure ulcer:** Any lesion caused by unrelieved pressure resulting in damage of underlying tissue.

**Prone:** Lying face downward.

**Pseudotumor cerebri:** A condition whose symptoms mirror those of a brain tumor: increased intracranial pressure, headache, nausea, brief periods of vision loss (graying or blurring) and double vision. The cause is unknown, but patients are often obese women.

**Pulsed lavage:** A form of mechanical debridement using intermittent or pulsed jets of irrigant and simultaneous suction to debride a wound.

**Renin:** An enzyme released by the kidney to help control the body's sodium-potassium balance, fluid volume, and blood pressure.

**Reverse Trendelenburg position:** Lying supine with head higher than the pelvis.

**Roux-en-Y:** Also known as gastric bypass. Surgeons divide a patient's stomach into a smaller pouch and re-route the intestine to effect malabsorption.

**Serotonin transporter:** A monoamine transporter protein that allows neurons, platelets, and other cells to accumulate the chemical neurotransmitter serotonin, which affects emotions and drives.

**Severe obesity:** A designation given to those persons whose BMI is over 40.

**Sibutramine:** A common prescription appetite suppressant, it is sold under the brand name Meridia.

**Sleep apnea:** Cessation of breathing for 10 or more seconds during sleep.

**Super obesity:** Also known as morbid obesity, is a designation given to those persons whose BMI is over 40.

**Supine:** Lying flat on back, with face upward.

**Syndrome X:** An older phrase describing a combination of health conditions that place a person at high risk for heart disease. Now referred to as metabolic syndrome.

**Thrifty gene:** Refers to a theory that due to an adaptation to the environment from former times when food was only available a few times a year, certain groups of people do not have built-in appetite suppressants. When food became available, these people were able to eat more and store more fat in order to sur-

vive the months when food was not readily available.

**Tidal volume:** The amount (volume) of air inhaled and exhaled with each normal breath.

**Tracheostomy:** Surgery to create an opening (stoma) into the windpipe. The opening itself may also be called a tracheostomy.

**Transferrin:** A type of protein that acts as the vehicle for transporting iron between different sites in the body.

**Type 1 diabetes (or insulin-dependent diabetes):** Occurs when the pancreas is unable to produce insulin. It is caused by the destruction of the beta cells in the pancreas by the body's immune system. It usually develops in childhood or adolescence but may appear at any age. Insulin administration is required.

**Type 2 diabetes (or non-insulin-dependent diabetes):** Occurs when the pancreas does not produce enough insulin to meet the body's needs or the insulin is not metabolized effectively. Type 2 diabetes is usually treated through diet and exercise, although some people must also take oral medications or insulin.

**Venous disease:** A variety of conditions affecting the legs, including deep vein thrombosis (DVT), venous stasis disease, phlebitis, and varicose veins.

**Vertical banded gastroplasty:** A surgical procedure that involves stapling the stomach to reduce its size to a thumb-sized pouch. The outlet to the pouch is reinforced with a synthetic mesh band. The result is a marked restriction in the volume of food that can be consumed, inducing the feeling of satiety after only a few bites. Also known as "Stomach Stapling" or "Gastric Stapling."

**Visceral fat:** One of the three compartments of abdominal fat.

**Vital capacity:** The amount of air that can be breathed out after taking the largest possible breath.

**Weight cycling:** The repeated loss and regain of body weight. When weight cycling is the result of dieting, it is often called "yo-yo" dieting.

**Weight Watchers:** Weight Watchers, founded in the 1960s, is a company offering various dieting products and services to assist in weight loss.

**Yeast infection:** Another term for candidiasis infection.